Observational Gait Analysis

A Visual Guide

Observational Gait Analysis

A Visual Guide

Janet M. Adams, PT, MS, DPT
Professor
Department of Physical Therapy
California State University, Northridge
Northridge, California

Kay Cerny, PT, PhD
Professor Emeritus
Department of Physical Therapy
California State University, Long Beach
Long Beach, California

Illustrator: Daniel Sanchez, PT

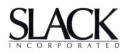

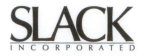

SLACK Incorporated
6900 Grove Road
Thorofare, NJ 08086 USA
856-848-1000   Fax: 856-848-6091
www.Healio.com/books
© 2018 by SLACK Incorporated

Senior Vice President: Stephanie Portnoy
Vice President, Editorial: Jennifer Kilpatrick
Vice President, Marketing: Michelle Gatt
Acquisitions Editor: Tony Schiavo
Managing Editor: Allegra Tiver
Creative Director: Thomas Cavallaro
Cover Artist: Christine Seabo
Project Editor: Erin O'Reilly

Observational Gait Analysis: A Visual Guide includes ancillary materials specifically available for faculty use. Please visit http://www.efacultylounge.com to obtain access.

The procedures and practices described in this publication should be implemented in a manner consistent with the professional standards set for the circumstances that apply in each specific situation. Every effort has been made to confirm the accuracy of the information presented and to correctly relate generally accepted practices. The authors, editors, and publisher cannot accept responsibility for errors or exclusions or for the outcome of the material presented herein. There is no expressed or implied warranty of this book or information imparted by it. Care has been taken to ensure that drug selection and dosages are in accordance with currently accepted/recommended practice. Off-label uses of drugs may be discussed. Due to continuing research, changes in government policy and regulations, and various effects of drug reactions and interactions, it is recommended that the reader carefully review all materials and literature provided for each drug, especially those that are new or not frequently used. Some drugs or devices in this publication have clearance for use in a restricted research setting by the Food and Drug and Administration or FDA. Each professional should determine the FDA status of any drug or device prior to use in their practice.

Any review or mention of specific companies or products is not intended as an endorsement by the author or publisher.

SLACK Incorporated uses a review process to evaluate submitted material. Prior to publication, educators or clinicians provide important feedback on the content that we publish. We welcome feedback on this work.

Library of Congress Cataloging-in-Publication Data

Names: Adams, Janet M., author. | Cerny, Kay, author.
Title: Observational gait analysis : a visual guide / Janet M. Adams, Kay
   Cerny.
Description: Thorofare, NJ : SLACK Incorporated, [2018] | Includes
   bibliographical references and index.
Identifiers: LCCN 2017043247 (print) | LCCN 2017044472 (ebook) | ISBN
   9781630910426 (Web) | ISBN 9781630910419 (Epub) | ISBN 9781630910402 (alk.
   paper)
Subjects: | MESH: Gait--physiology | Kinetics | Atlases
Classification: LCC QP303 (ebook) | LCC QP303 (print) | NLM WE 17 | DDC
   612.7/6--dc23

For permission to reprint material in another publication, contact SLACK Incorporated. Authorization to photocopy items for internal, personal, or academic use is granted by SLACK Incorporated provided that the appropriate fee is paid directly to Copyright Clearance Center. Prior to photocopying items, please contact the Copyright Clearance Center at 222 Rosewood Drive, Danvers, MA 01923 USA; phone: 978-750-8400; website: www.copyright.com; email: info@copyright.com

Printed in the United States of America.

Last digit is print number: 10   9   8   7   6   5   4   3   2

DEDICATIONS

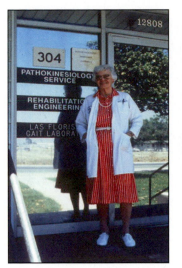

Jacquelin Perry, MD

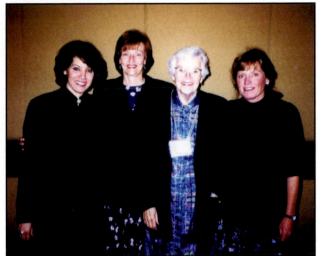

Left to right: Dr. Olfat Mohamed, Dr. Kay Cerny, Dr. Jacquelin Perry, and Dr. Janet M. Adams

DEDICATED TO JACQUELIN PERRY, MD (MAY 31, 1918—MARCH 11, 2013)

Dedicated with gratitude to an extraordinary mentor, researcher, and clinician—Jacquelin Perry, MD—whose passion for scientific inquiry and evidence-based medicine enhanced the lives of numerous patients, students, clinicians, and academicians.

One month before Dr. Perry's death at the age of 94, we (Drs. Adams and Cerny) spoke with her at an American Physical Therapy Association conference about writing a new pedagogical text to teach observational gait analysis. She expressed support for its concept and offered to work on the text with us. We were to meet in April 2013, but she passed away just weeks before our meeting. We would like to think that Dr. Perry is guiding us on this project, and we express our sincere thanks for both her willingness to work on this text with us and her mentorship over the course of our careers.

Janet M. Adams' Dedication

Dedicated to my father Rex McNaught Adams, a mechanical engineer who, by example, instilled in me a strong work ethic, attention to detail, and pride in a job well done. To my mother Marianna Helena Adams, a kindhearted and generous humanitarian who has supported the efforts of many. To my dear friends, Joyce Griffin and Lawrence Lovell, for their steadfast support and friendship. A special thanks to my good friends, colleagues, and coauthors Kay Cerny and Olfat Mohamed for their dedication and perseverance in making this text a reality. And to Dr. Perry for her mentorship and high level of expectation throughout my career.

Kay Cerny's Dedication

Dedicated to my family for their on-going love and support over the years: to my father who helped me learn compassion for the planet and all living things; to my mother who helped me learn that respect is earned; and to my brother, Chuck, who is forever dear to my heart for his child-like goodness. To Edna Daufen, for her true friendship since physical therapy school. To Dr. Perry, for expecting that I practice the highest level of physical therapy at Rancho Los Amigos. To Olfat Mohamed for providing a thorough review of functional measures important to gait. To Jan Adams for inviting me to coauthor this book: only through her steadfast determination did we see this text come to fruition.

CONTENTS

▶ Section II   Case Studies 171

Section III   Appendices 211

Observational Gait Analysis: A Visual Guide includes ancillary materials specifically available for faculty use. Please visit http://www.efacultylounge.com to obtain access.

Acknowledgments

Both authors wish to extend a special thanks to two individuals whose technical expertise made this text possible. To Daniel Sanchez, a former physical therapy student at California State University, Northridge, for his diligence, creativity, and attentiveness in creating beautiful illustrations that truly make this text a "visual guide." To Matthew David Sandusky, biomedical engineer, for his technical expertise, and support in maintaining and advancing the Pathokinesiology Laboratory at California State University, Long Beach where the Vicon recording and videotaping took place.

The authors also wish to thank the following colleagues for their support:

Leslie Torburn, PT, DPT
Physical Therapist
Motion Analysis Center
Shriners Hospital for Children Northern California
Sacramento, California

Kristin DeMars, PT, DPT, NCS
Lecturer
Department of Physical Therapy
California State University, Long Beach
Long Beach, California

Sheryl Low, PT, DPT, DSc, PCS,
Department Chair and Professor
Department of Physical Therapy
California State University, Northridge
Northridge, California

Courtney Peterson, SPT
Department of Physical Therapy
California State University, Northridge
Northridge, California

Sculpture on book cover "Astride-Aside" by artist Michael Stutz
Located at South Pasadena Mission Street Plaza
Dedicated February 22, 2003
"It represents a celebration of everyday life, emphasizing movement and direction in an ever-changing urban world. By placing the walking man sculpture on blocks from the Sante Fe Historic Bridge, the work literally builds upon on the foundation of the past."—*Michael Stutz*

Similarly, *Observational Gait Analysis: A Visual Guide*, builds on the past work of many clinicians, especially that of Dr. Jacquelin Perry, Dr. Verne Inman, and Dr. David Sutherland who built the scientific foundation for clinical gait analysis.

ABOUT THE AUTHORS

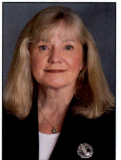

Janet M. Adams, PT, MS, DPT earned her bachelor's degree in Physical Therapy from the University of Illinois in Chicago in 1976. She began her physical therapy career specializing in pediatrics at Spalding School for Handicapped Children (Chicago, Illinois) until 1978 when she moved to Phoenix, Arizona where she was the Director of the Physical Therapy Department at Gompers Rehabilitation Center. In 1980, following her move to Los Angeles, California she began her master of science degree at University of Southern California (USC) and began working with Dr. Jacquelin Perry at the Pathokinesiology Service at Rancho Los Amigos National Rehabilitation Center (Downey, California). Dr. Adams earned both her master of science and doctorate of Physical Therapy at USC. In 1992, Dr. Adams began her career in academia at California State University, Northridge (CSUN) where she has taught for over 25 years. Currently, Dr. Adams is a full-time tenured professor in the Department of Physical Therapy at CSUN and a Research Associate at California State University, Long Beach (CSULB) where she works on doctoral research projects with Dr. Cerny. Dr. Adams has taught classes in applied biomechanics, normal and pathological gait analysis, prosthetics and orthotics, applied anatomy, evidence based practice, and research design and methodology. She supervises doctoral research students at both CSUN and CSULB. In addition to numerous publications, Dr. Adams has authored 2 chapters with Dr. Perry in 2 editions of Verne Inman's text *Human Walking*.

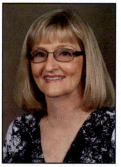

Kay Cerny, PT, PhD earned her bachelor's degree from Miami University (Oxford, Ohio). She received her certificate in Physical Therapy from the D.T Watson School of Physiatrics (Leetsdale, Pennsylvania) in 1963. Dr. Cerny began her clinical practice at Rancho Los Amigos National Rehabilitation Center, and was one of the original physical therapists who worked with Dr. Jacquelin Perry on developing observational gait analysis (OGA) for clinicians and helped author the first edition of the Rancho OGA manual. She was one of the traveling Rancho therapists who introduced the then-new approach of clinical gait analysis to physical therapists across the country and Canada in the early 1970s.

At Rancho, Dr. Cerny planned, wrote, and executed teaching materials for physical therapy staff, interns, and aides. Her part-time teaching included kinesiology for orthotic-prosthetic students at Cerritos College (Cerritos, California). In 1969, she took a 1-year leave from Rancho to teach physical therapy students full time at the University of Texas, Medical Branch in Galveston. Returning to Rancho, she soon transferred to the Pathokinesiology Service to evaluate patients with Dr. Perry. Dr. Cerny earned her master of science in Physical Therapy from the University of Southern California (Los Angeles) studying walking and wheelchair energetics in people with paraplegia secondary to spinal cord injury.

In 1978, Dr. Cerny accepted a full-time position teaching physical therapy at California State University, Northridge. Four years later, after earning tenure, she accepted a tenure-track position at California State University, Long Beach (CSULB), where she earned tenure and advanced to full professor. At CSULB, she taught applied biomechanics, including normal and pathological gait, and supported student research projects that have resulted in subsequent peer-reviewed publications. In 2004, she accepted the Department Chair position, which she held from 2004 until 2014. Under her chairmanship, the Department of Physical Therapy advanced to the DPT program, began an out patient faculty practice, and was successfully reaccredited. She earned her PhD from the University of Southern California in 1987 where she studied the effect of simulated knee flexion contractures on gait. Dr. Cerny retired in 2015 to limit her teaching to supervising DPT student research and to assist in writing this text.

CONTRIBUTING AUTHOR

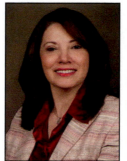

Olfat Mohamed, PT, PhD is a full-time tenured professor in the Department of Physical Therapy at California State University, Long Beach. Dr. Mohamed earned her bachelor's dgree in Physical Therapy from Cairo University, Egypt, in 1974. Because of her excellent academic achievements, she was appointed by the University as an instructor at the Faculty of Physical Therapy, immediately after her graduation from the bachelor's program. In addition to her academic responsibilities, Dr. Mohamed practiced physical therapy in several of Cairo's University hospitals. She earned her master of science degree in Physical Therapy in 1979 from Cairo University as well. Dr. Mohamed traveled to several countries for teaching and clinical duties. In 1983, she was awarded a full scholarship from the Egyptian Government to pursue her doctorate degree. Dr. Mohamed moved to Los Angeles, California and joined the doctoral program at the University of Southern California (USC) where she earned her PhD in Physical Therapy in 1989. She performed her doctorate and postdoctorate research with Dr. Jacquelin Perry at the Pathokinesiology Service at Rancho Los Amigos National Rehabilitation Center. Dr. Mohamed publishes and presents both nationally and internationally on gait and balance disorders. She is also a curriculum consultant and a visiting professor at Cairo University.

INTRODUCTION

Our intent in compiling this manual is to address all aspects of analyzing walking in one comprehensive teaching text. Since observational gait analysis (OGA) is an acquired skill requiring practice and feedback, we have included videos of persons with and without gait deviations for the student and clinician to observe.

The manual begins with the most necessary and simple calculation of walking speed and its functional significance, then delves into temporal and spatial characteristics in the normal population as a basis for comparison with persons with disabilities. The student is next introduced to kinematics with illustrations and descriptions of sagittal plane motion as well as frontal and transverse motions. Kinetics are then introduced with visualization of the ground reaction force vector superimposed on the figures, providing a basis for understanding external moments and the associated demands placed on muscles and passive structures.

With an emphasis on "functional assessment" in today's health care environment, the chapter on functional tools and their psychometric properties is invaluable. The combination of Chapters 1 through 5 will enhance the student's ability to integrate the association between the *International Classification of Functioning, Disability and Health* (ICF) domains of body function (impairments), activity, and participation measures.

A newly developed OGA form addresses major gait deviations and their likely occurrence in the gait cycle. Deviations are defined in the manual and linked with video clips to enhance the student's observational skills. The probable cause(s) of each deviation are separated into primary, secondary, and compensatory causes. Students can then plan and perform the clinical evaluation of their patients to verify probable primary and secondary causes and differentiate them from useful compensatory strategies.

Lastly, the authors performed 7 case studies that require the student to read the history and evaluation results from the patient report, view multiple videos of the patient walking, identify deviations, and complete the newly developed OGA form. To complete the OGA form, the student has access to the main videos as well as Vicon Polygon films, which include videos taken simultaneously with an instrumented gait analysis. The videos include anterior-posterior and lateral views of the patient, a skeletal model of the patient walking, and kinematic and kinetic graphs in real time and slow motion (50%).

Instructors can compare the student's OGA assessment and 3 expert examiners' results by accessing the SLACK Incorporated efaculty lounge (website available to faculty only). Instructors also can review the final report generated by the expert examiners, also located on the efaculty lounge website.

Our intent was to centrally locate all the *necessary* material to enhance the student's learning of observational gait analysis in a single text. We hope that this manual compliments the text by Perry and Burnfield, which was the major source for the material.

As Dr. Adams has taught and practiced gait analysis for over 40 years and Dr. Cerny for over 50 years, we realized that a more comprehensive teaching manual/text was needed to assist the student in learning observational gait analysis. The intent of this manual is to provide a visual guide for observational analysis with improved illustrations, videos, and case studies to enhance student problem solving. This manual/text is intended to accompany and compliment Drs. Perry and Burnfield's text *Normal & Pathological Gait* also published by SLACK Incorporated.

I

Normal and Pathological Gait

Chapter 1

Walking Speed
The Sixth Vital Sign

When evaluating a client's functional abilities, walking speed or gait velocity should be measured as it is a key indicator of function. It can be appreciated as the 6th vital sign[1,2] as it reflects the general function of the cardiorespiratory, musculoskeletal, and neurological systems, and the health of the individual by comparison with established normative values.[3-6] Vital signs 1 through 5 include pulse rate, respiratory rate, blood pressure, pain, and temperature.

Walking speed is measured routinely and has established reliability and validity,[7] predicts functional participation,[5,6,8] health status,[9] cognitive impairments,[10] and mortality.[11] A task force from the International Academy on Nutrition & Aging found that walking speed identified autonomous community-dwelling older people at risk for adverse outcomes and recommended it be used as a single-item assessment tool.[12] Measuring walking speed is safe, quick, cost-effective, and easy to measure in almost any environment.

1.1: DETERMINANTS OF WALKING SPEED

A person can increase walking speed by either increasing the number of steps taken per minute and/or by increasing the length of his or her stride. Walking speed (velocity) is the product of stride length (m) and ½ cadence (steps/min).

Walking Speed (Velocity): The distance traversed during a specified time period (m/sec or m/min).

Normal Adult[3]
Men: 82 m/min or 1.37 m/sec
Women: 78 m/min or 1.30 m/sec

Cadence: The number of steps taken during a specified time period (steps/min).

Normal Adult[3]
Men: 108 steps/min
Women: 118 steps/min

Stride Length: The linear distance between 2 successive events (Initial Contact in normal gait) on the same limb.

Example: Right heel contact to right heel contact
Normal Adult[3]
Men: 1.51 m
Women: 1.32 m

Adams JM, Cerny K.
Observational Gait Analysis: A Visual Guide (pp 3-8).
© 2018 SLACK Incorporated.

1.2: MEASURING WALKING SPEED, CADENCE, AND STRIDE LENGTH: 10-METER WALK TEST

1. Mark off 10 m (6 m for data collection, bounded by 2 m for acceleration and 2 m for deceleration)
2. Determine the time it takes to traverse the 6 m (stopwatch/cell phone)
3. Count the steps (both left and right) taken in the 6 m area

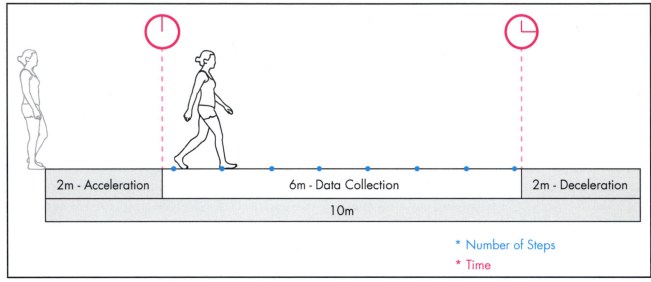

Figure 1-1. Walkway for measuring velocity, cadence, and stride length.

   Example: You instructed your patient to walk at a self-selected pace over a 10-m walkway. Within the central 6 m, you count 8 steps taken over 5 seconds. Calculate the walking speed, cadence, and stride length.

Walking Speed (Velocity) = Distance ÷ Time

Walking Speed = 6 m ÷ 5 sec = **1.2 m/sec x** (60 sec/min) = **72 m/min**

Cadence = Steps ÷ Time

Cadence = 8 steps ÷ 5 sec x (60 sec/min) = **96 steps/min**
Walking speed = stride length x ½ cadence

Stride Length = Walking Speed ÷ ½ Cadence

Stride length = 72 m/min ÷ (1/2 x 96 step/min) = 48 strides/min = **1.5 m/stride**

1.3: NORMAL VALUES FOR ADULTS AGES 20 TO 59 YEARS OLD

Self-Selected Walking Speed

TABLE 1-1		
WOMEN **M/SEC (M/MIN)**	**MEN** **M/SEC (M/MIN)**	**REFERENCES**
1.30 m/sec (77.7 m/min)	1.37 m/sec (82.0 m/min)	Waters et al[3] (n = 34 women, 39 men)
1.32 m/sec (79.3 m/min)	1.36 m/sec (82.1 m/min)	Rancho Los Amigos National Rehabilitation Center[4] (n = 129 women, 109 men)
1.27 m/sec (76.2 m/min)	1.34 m/sec (80.4 m/min)	Kadaba et al[5] (n = 12 women, 28 men)
1.40 m/sec (84.1 m/min)	1.43 m/sec (85.6 m/min)	Bohannon[6] (n = 87 women, 87 men)
Reference values for self-selected pace/comfortable walking speed		

Self-Selected Cadence and Stride Length

TABLE 1-2			
	WOMEN	**MEN**	**REFERENCES**
STRIDE LENGTH	**Meters**	**Meters**	
	1.32	1.51	Waters et al[3]
	1.32	1.48	Rancho Los Amigos National Rehabilitation Center[4]
	1.30	1.41	Kadaba et al[5]
CADENCE	**Steps/Min**	**Steps/Min**	
	118	108	Waters et al[3]
	121	111	Rancho Los Amigos National Rehabilitation Center[4]
	115	112	Kadaba et al[5]
Reference values for cadence and stride length at self-selected pace/comfortable walking speed			

1.4: MEANINGFUL CHANGE IN WALKING SPEED

A *meaningful change* reflects actual differences that are attributed to true patient improvement rather than measurement error. There are 2 psychometric properties that have been derived for outcome tools.

Minimal Detectable Change

The minimal detectable change (MDC) is the smallest change that reflects a *true* difference above measurement error (eg, standard error of the mean).

Minimal Clinically Important Difference

The minimal clinically important difference (MCID) is the difference perceived to be functionally significant by the patient or expert clinician.[13]

TABLE 1-3. MDC AND MCID OF SPEED FOR MULTIPLE DIAGNOSTIC GROUPS			
DIAGNOSTIC GROUP	**MDC (M/SEC)**	**MCID (M/SEC)**	**REFERENCES**
Hip fractures	0.17	——	Latham et al[14]
	0.08	0.10	Palombaro et al[15]
Parkinson's	0.18	——	Steffen and Seney[16]
Multiple sclerosis	——	>20% of initial speed	Hobart et al[17]
	——	0.11	Coleman et al[18]
Spinal cord injury	0.13	0.13	Lam et al[19]
Stroke (in-patient)	——	0.13	Bohannon et al[20]
Stroke (out-patient)	——	0.175	Fulk et al[21]
Stroke (out-patient)	——	0.16	Tilson et al[22]
Elderly adults	——	0.10	Perera et al[23]

1.5: WALKING SPEED AND FUNCTIONAL PARTICIPATION CATEGORIES

Perry[8] found that patients with stroke who were categorized in these functional participation walking categories achieved these average walking speeds.

TABLE 1-4		
FUNCTIONAL CATEGORY	**SPEED**	
NORMAL WALKING SPEED	1.37 m/sec	(82 m/min)
Physiological Walker	0.1 m/sec	(6 m/min)
Limited Household Walker	0.23 m/sec	(13.8 m/min)
Unlimited Household Walker	0.27 m/sec	(16.2 m/min)
Most-Limited Community Walker	0.4 m/sec	(24 m/min)
Unlimited Community Walker	0.8 m/sec	(48 m/min)

1.6: FUNCTIONAL PARTICIPATION WALKING CATEGORIES: CLASSIFICATION OF WALKING HANDICAP (BASED ON PATIENTS WITH STROKE)[8]

Physiological Walker

- Walks for exercise at home or in parallel bars

Limited Household Walker

- Relies on walking to some extent for home activities
- Requires assistance for some walking activities, uses a wheelchair, or is unable to perform others

Unlimited Household Walker

- Able to use walking for all household activities without any reliance on a wheelchair
- Encounters difficulty with stairs and uneven terrain
- May not be able to enter and leave the house independently

Most-Limited Community Walker

- Can enter and leave the house independently
- Can ascend and descend curbs independently and stairs to some degree
- Independent in at least one moderate community activity (appointments or restaurants)
- Unable or needs assistance in no more than one other low-challenge activity (eg, church, neighborhood, visiting a friend)

Least-Limited Community Walker

- Independent on ascending and descending stairs
- Independent in all moderate community activities without assistance or a wheelchair
- Independent in either local stores or uncrowded shopping centers

Unlimited Community Walker

- Independent in all home and community activities
- Can navigate crowds and uneven terrain independently
- Demonstrates complete independence in shopping centers

1.7: References

1. Fritz S, Lusardi M. White paper: "walking speed: the sixth vital sign." *J Geriatr Phys Ther.* 2009;32(2):46-49.
2. Middleton A, Fritz SL, Lusardi M. Walking speed: the functional vital sign. *J Aging Phys Act.* 2015;23(2):314-322.
3. Waters RL, Lunsford BR, Perry J, Byrd R. Energy-speed relationship of walking: standard tables. *J Orthop Res.* 1988;6(2):215-222.
4. Pathokinesiology Service & the Physical Therapy Department. *Observational Gait Analysis.* 4th ed. Rancho Los Amigos National Rehabilitaton Center, Downey, CA: Los Amigos Research and Educational Institute Inc; 2001.
5. Kadaba MP, Ramakrishnan HK, Wootten ME. Measurement of lower extremity kinematics during level walking. *J Orthop Res.* 1990;8(3):383-392.
6. Bohannon RW. Comfortable and maximum walking speed of adults aged 20-79 years: reference values and determinants. *Age Ageing.* 1997;26(1):15-19.
7. Steffen TM, Hacker TA, Mollinger L. Age- and gender-related test performance in community-dwelling elderly people: Six-Minute Walk Test, Berg Balance Scale, Timed Up & Go Test, and gait speeds. *Phys Ther.* 2002;82(2):128-137.
8. Perry J, Garrett M, Gronley JK, Mulroy SJ. Classification of walking handicap in the stroke population. *Stroke.* 1995;26(6):982-989.
9. Purser JL, Weinberger M, Cohen HJ, et al. Walking speed predicts health status and hospital costs for frail elderly male veterans. *J Rehabil Res Dev.* 2005;42(4):535-546.
10. Bridenbaugh SA, Kressig RW. Quantitative gait disturbances in older adults with cognitive impairments. *Curr Pharm Des.* 2014;20(19):3165-3172.
11. Hardy SE, Perera S, Roumani YF, Chandler JM, Studenski SA. Improvement in usual gait speed predicts better survival in older adults. *J Am Geriatr Soc.* 2007;55(11):1727-1734.
12. Abellan van Kan G, Rolland Y, Andrieu S, et al. Gait speed at usual pace as a predictor of adverse outcomes in community-dwelling older people an International Academy on Nutrition and Aging (IANA) Task Force. *J Nutr Health Aging.* 2009;13(10):881-889.
13. Beaton DE, Boers M, Wells GA. Many faces of the minimal clinically important difference (MCID): a literature review and directions for future research. *Curr Opin Rheumatol.* 2002;14(2):109-114.
14. Latham NK, Mehta V, Nguyen AM, et al. Performance-based or self-report measures of physical function: which should be used in clinical trials of hip fracture patients? *Arch Phys Med Rehabil.* 2008;89(11):2146-2155.
15. Palombaro KM, Craik RL, Mangione KK, Tomlinson JD. Determining meaningful changes in gait speed after hip fracture. *Phys Ther.* 2006;86(6):809-816.
16. Steffen T, Seney M. Test-retest reliability and minimal detectable change on balance and ambulation tests, the 36-item short-form health survey, and the unified Parkinson disease rating scale in people with parkinsonism. *Phys Ther.* 2008;88(6):733-746.
17. Hobart J, Blight AR, Goodman A, Lynn F, Putzki N. Timed 25-foot walk: direct evidence that improving 20% or greater is clinically meaningful in MS. *Neurology.* 2013;80(16):1509-1517.
18. Coleman CI, Sobieraj DM, Marinucci LN. Minimally important clinical difference of the timed 25-foot walk test: results from a randomized controlled trial in patients with multiple sclerosis. *Curr Med Res Opin.* 2012;28(1):49-56.
19. Lam T, Noonan VK, Eng JJ. A systematic review of functional ambulation outcome measures in spinal cord injury. *Spinal Cord.* 2008;46(4):246-254.
20. Bohannon RW, Andrews AW, Glenney SS. Minimal clinically important difference for comfortable speed as a measure of gait performance in patients undergoing inpatient rehabilitation after stroke. *J Phys Ther Sci.* 2013;25(10):1223-1225.
21. Fulk GD, Ludwig M, Dunning K, Golden S, Boyne P, West T. Estimating clinically important change in gait speed in people with stroke undergoing outpatient rehabilitation. *J Neurol Phys Ther.* 2011;35(2):82-89.
22. Tilson JK, Sullivan KJ, Cen SY, et al. Meaningful gait speed improvement during the first 60 days poststroke: minimal clinically important difference. *Phys Ther.* 2010;90(2):196-208.
23. Perera S, Mody SH, Woodman RC, Studenski SA. Meaningful change and responsiveness in common physical performance measures in older adults. *J Am Geriatr Soc.* 2006;54(5):743-749.

Chapter 2

Temporal and Spatial Gait Characteristics

2.1: TIMING (TEMPORAL) CHARACTERISTICS

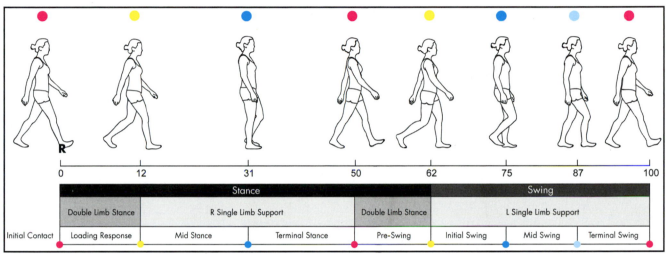

Figure 2-1. Temporal characteristics (right lower extremity [LE] is the reference limb).

Gait Cycle (GC): The time from Initial Contact to Initial Contact on the same foot including both stance phase and swing phase.

> ie, right foot Initial Contact to right foot Initial Contact
> **Normal Adult: (~ 1 sec from 0% to 100% GC)[1]**

Stance Phase: The time when the foot is in contact with the support surface during one gait cycle.

> ie, right foot Initial Contact to right foot toe-off
> **Normal Adult: 0.62 sec (62% GC)[1]**
> **Occurs from 0% to 62% GC**

Single Limb Support (SLS): The time when only one foot is in contact with the support surface during one gait cycle.

> ie, right foot SLS is initiated by left toe-off and ends at left foot Initial Contact (by definition when the left foot is airborne, the right foot is in SLS).
> **Normal Adult: 0.38 sec (38% GC)[1]**
> **Occurs from 12% to 50% GC**

Adams JM, Cerny K.
Observational Gait Analysis: A Visual Guide (pp 9-19).
© 2018 SLACK Incorporated.

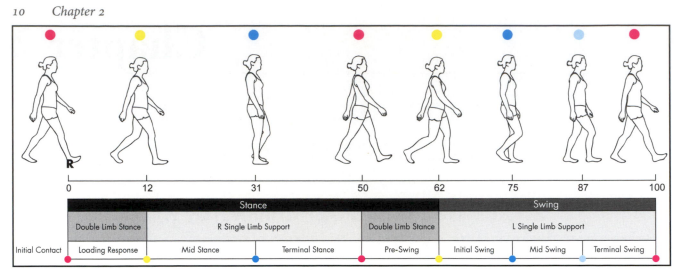

Figure 2-1. Temporal characteristics (right LE is the reference limb).

Double Limb Stance (DLS): The time when both feet are in contact with the support surface during one gait cycle. Weight transfer is occurring between the limbs.

ie, right limb is undergoing Loading Response, while left limb is being unloaded in Pre-Swing (both feet are in contact with the ground).
Normal Adult: 0.24 sec (24% GC)

Initial Double Limb Stance (Loading Response): The time when the support limb is undergoing Loading Response.

ie, right foot Initial Contact and ends at left foot toe-off
Initial DLS from 0% to 12% GC[1]

Terminal Double Limb Stance (Pre-Swing): The time when the support limb is being unloaded.

ie, left foot Initial Contact to right foot toe-off
Terminal DLS from 50% to 62% GC[1]

Swing Phase: The time when the foot is airborne during one gait cycle.

ie, right foot toe-off to right foot Initial Contact
Normal Adult: 0.38 sec (38% GC)[1]
Occurs from 62% to 100% GC

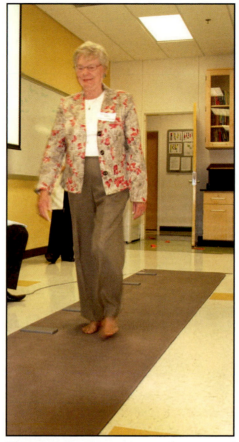

Figure 2-2. Assessment of temporal and spatial gait characteristics using the GaitRite System (CIR Systems, Inc).

Gender	Age	Left - Leg - Right		
M	38	89	89	

Long Gap 2 (Toe In/Out) — Pattern↓ — Unassisted ↓ FAP **68**

Bilateral Parameters	Left	Right
→ Step Time (sec)	.69	.95
→ Cycle Time (sec)	1.64	1.32
Step Length (cm)	81.92	71.02
Stride Length (cm)	153.34	157.92
H-H Base Support (cm)	10.52	5.09
→ Single Support (%GC)	27.4	36.1
→ Double Support (%GC)	20.4	27.6
→ Swing (%GC)	29.1	34.1
→ Stance (%GC)	70.9	65.9
Step/Extremity Ratio	.92	.80
Toe In / Out (deg)	2	12

Parameters	
Distance (cm)	305.9
Ambulation Time (sec)	3.27
Velocity (cm/sec)	93.5
Mean Normalized Velocity	1.05
Number of Steps	4
Cadence (Steps/Min)	73.4
Step Time Differential (sec)	.26
Step Length Differential (cm)	10.90
Cycle Time Differential (sec)	.32

Prim Dr [Johnson] — Problem [L hip pain] — [Samp

Figure 2-3. A printout of the temporal and spatial gait characteristics using the GaitRite System (CIR Systems, Inc).

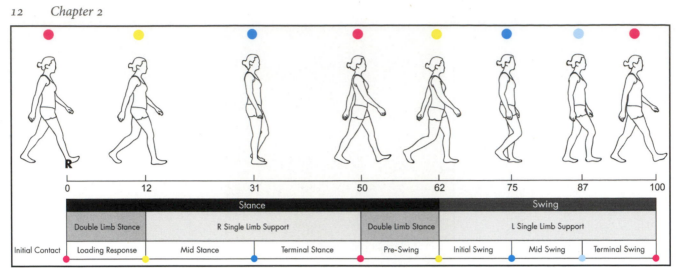

Figure 2-1. Temporal characteristics (right LE is the reference limb).

2.2: Stance Phase: 0% to 62% Gait Cycle (Right Lower Extremity Is the Reference Limb)

● Initial Contact (0% to 2% GC)

The instant when the foot contacts the support surface; heel contact normally occurs. The first pink circle marks Initial Contact.

● Loading Response (2% to 12% GC)

The first interval of DLS (initial DLS) when weight is transferred to the supporting limb. The contralateral (CL) limb is being unloaded (CL Pre-Swing). The first yellow circle marks the end of Loading Response at 12% GC.

● Mid Stance (12% to 31% GC)

The first half of single limb support (SLS) is initiated by (CL) limb toe-off. The center of mass (COM) progresses dynamic stability over a plantigrade foot. The turquoise circle marks the end of Mid Stance at 31% GC.

● Terminal Stance (31% to 50% GC)

The second half of SLS. The COM continues to progress anterior to the ankle joint axis toward the metatarsal axis. Heel rise normally occurs during this phase at ~ 34% GC.[2] The second pink circle marks the end of Terminal Stance at 50% GC.

● Pre-Swing (50% to 62% GC)

The second interval of DLS when the support limb is unloaded in preparation for swing and weight is transferred to the CL limb (initiated by Initial Contact of the CL limb). The second yellow circle marks the end of Pre-Swing at 62% GC.

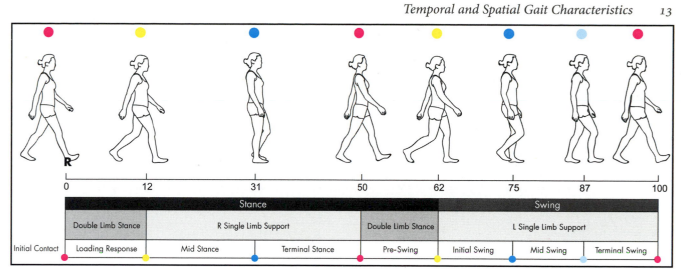

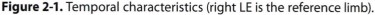

Figure 2-1. Temporal characteristics (right LE is the reference limb).

2.3: SWING PHASE: 62% TO 100% GAIT CYCLE (RIGHT LOWER EXTREMITY IS THE REFERENCE LIMB)

Swing is divided equally into 3 phases. Right foot swing phase is initiated by right toe-off and ends at right foot Initial Contact.

● Initial Swing (62% to 75% GC)

The initial period of swing when the foot is lifted off the support surface (defined by ipsilateral toe-off), and the limb begins to advance forward. The CL limb is therefore in the first half of SLS (Mid Stance). The second turquoise circle marks the end of the Initial Swing at 75% GC.

○ Mid Swing (75% to 87% GC)

The midpoint of swing phase when minimal toe clearance (MTC) is achieved (at 81% GC), and the tibia reaches vertical in normal individuals. The CL limb is in late Mid Stance and early Terminal Stance. Note that tibial position should not be used to define Mid Swing in individuals with gait deviations. The light blue circle marks the end of Mid Swing at 87% GC.

● Terminal Swing (87% to 100% GC)

The final period of swing when the foot continues to advance forward in preparation for Initial Contact. The CL limb is in Terminal Stance. The last pink circle marks the end of Terminal Swing at 100% GC.

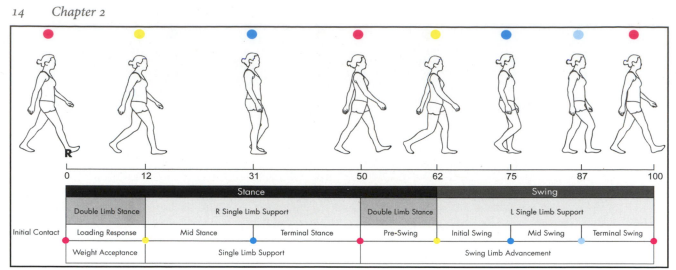

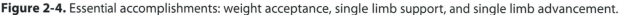

Figure 2-4. Essential accomplishments: weight acceptance, single limb support, and single limb advancement.

Essential Accomplishments: Essential accomplishments are those events that promote smooth forward progression and limb stability, with minimal excursion of the COM, conserving energy expenditure.

Weight Acceptance (0% to 12% GC)

Initial Contact

- Heel contact to advance COM forward (heel rocker)

Loading Response

- Controlled weight transfer to the stance limb
- Shock absorption

Single Limb Support (12% to 50% GC)

Mid Stance

- Dynamic stability over plantigrade foot as body weight is exclusively supported by a single limb
- Controlled forward progression of the COM from behind to in front of the ankle (ankle rocker)

Terminal Stance

- Dynamic stability over the forefoot as body weight is exclusively supported by a single limb
- Controlled forward progression of the COM anterior to foot with heel rise at ~ 34% GC[2] (forefoot rocker)

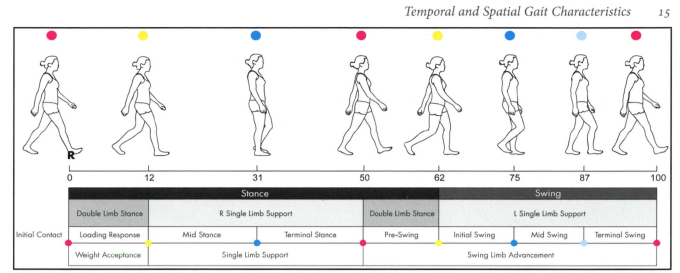

Figure 2-4. Essential accomplishments: weight acceptance, single limb support, and single limb advancement.

Essential Accomplishments (continued)

Swing Limb Advancement (50% to 100% GC)

Pre-Swing

- The thigh and knee flex in preparation for swing phase, weight is unloaded and transferred to the CL limb. This unweighting results in toe only contact (toe rocker).

Initial Swing

- Thigh advances forward
- Knee flexion achieves toe clearance

Mid Swing

- Thigh continues advancing
- Ankle dorsiflexes to neutral for toe clearance

Terminal Swing

- Knee extends to prepare for heel contact

2.4: Distance (Spatial) Characteristics

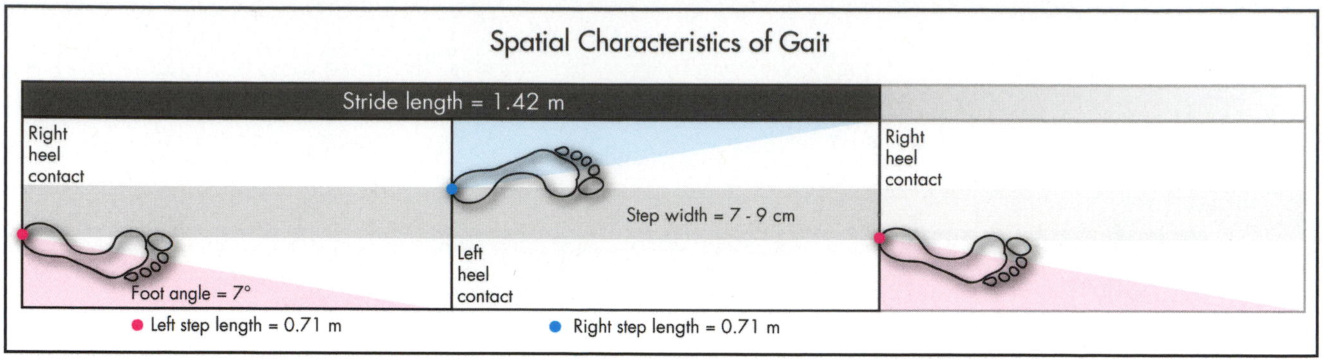

Figure 2-5. Spatial characteristics.

Stride Length: The linear distance between 2 successive events (Initial Contact) on the same limb.

> ie, right heel contact to right heel contact
> **Normal Adult: 1.42 m (Men: 1.51 m; Women: 1.32 m)[3,4]**

Step Length: The linear distance between 2 successive events on opposite limbs.

> ie, left step length is defined as right heel contact to left heel contact
> **Normal Adult: 0.71 m[4]**

Step Width: The horizontal distance between 2 points on opposite limbs.

> ie, right heel midpoint to left heel midpoint at Initial Contact
> **Normal Adult: 7 to 10 cm[4-6]**

Foot Progression Angle: The angle between the longitudinal axis of the foot and the line of gait progression.

> **Normal Adult: 5 to 7 degrees[5-7]**

Toe Clearance: The minimal linear distance from the hallux to the floor during swing phase (MTC).

> **Normal Adult: 1.28 cm at 80% GC[8] (Mid Swing)**
> **1.9 cm at 81% GC[9] (Mid Swing)**

2.5: PRIMARY DETERMINANTS
MINIMIZING CENTER OF MASS DISPLACEMENT

Minimal displacement of the COM, both vertically and laterally, is optimal for smooth, efficient, forward progression. Minimizing its excursion conserves energy, increases efficiency, and reduces muscular effort. With increased energy expenditure, both activity and participation measures of function are affected (eg, 6-minute walk test). Please refer to Chapter 5 for activities and participation measures.

In 1953, Saunders et al,[10] originally identified 6 essential motions as *gait determinants,* which minimized energy expenditure by reducing the excursion of the COM. He included pelvic rotation (transverse plane), pelvic list/obliquity (frontal plane), stance phase knee flexion, foot mechanics, knee mechanics, and hip adduction.

In 2001, Kerrigan[11] reported that pelvic rotation had little effect on minimizing the COM displacement, while both Della Croce et al[12] and Kerrigan et al[13] suggested that heel rise be included as a significant gait determinant.

In 2014, Lin et al[14] identified that vertical COM excursion was minimized by stance phase knee flexion, and the interaction of the ankle and foot (plantar flexion, toe dorsiflexion). Pelvic obliquity (frontal plane) and hip adduction were also included as primary determinants that minimized lateral COM displacement.[14]

Vertical Center of Mass Displacement

When the COM excursion is excessive, it requires increased muscular effort reducing efficiency and functional walking ability. COM movement in normal individuals is actually quite small (1 to 2 inches) and barely perceptible. Orendurff et al[15] found that during normal walking at a comfortable speed there is a double sinusoidal vertical trajectory of the COM displacing, $\sim 4.89 \pm 1.03$ cm. It is highest during SLS (Mid Stance at 30% of the GC) and lowest during DLS (Loading Response and Pre-Swing at 5% and 55% of the GC, respectively). They found that faster speeds increase the vertical COM excursion.[15]

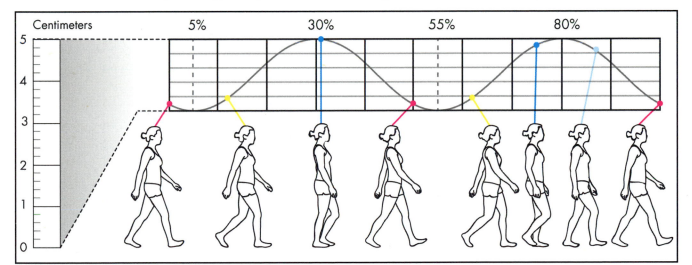

Figure 2-6. Vertical COM displacement during one GC (~ 5 cm). Note: Colored circles define phases.

Lateral Center of Mass Displacement

During normal walking at a comfortable speed there is a single sinusoidal lateral excursion of the COM of ~3.29±1.29 cm.[15] This displacement reflects the lateral shift of weight from one limb to another with maximum excursion in Mid Stance at 30% of the GC when weight is solely supported by the stance limb. The lateral shift is dependent on muscular stabilization of the hip and pelvis, so that pelvic drop and hip adduction are minimized.

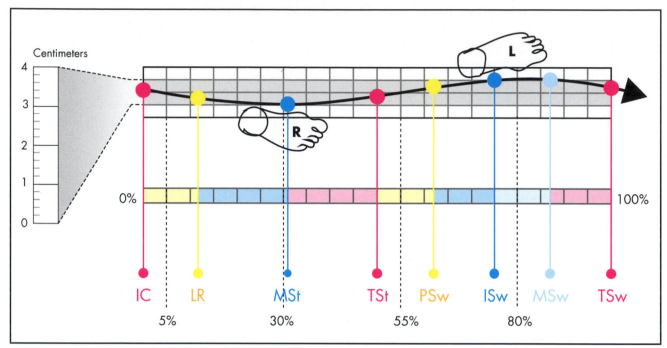

Figure 2-7. Lateral COM displacement during one GC (~4 cm). Note: colored circles define phases.

2.6: REFERENCES

1. Perry J, Burnfield JM. *Gait Analysis: Normal & Pathological Gait.* 2nd ed. Thorofare, NJ: SLACK Incorporated; 2010.
2. Bojsen-Moller F, Lamoreux L. Significance of free-dorsiflexion of the toes in walking. *Acta Orthop Scand.* 1979;50(4):471-479.
3. Waters RL, Lunsford BR, Perry J, Byrd R. Energy-speed relationship of walking: standard tables. *J Orthop Res.* 1988;6(2):215-222.
4. Marchetti GF, Whitney SL, Blatt PJ, Morris LO, Vance JM. Temporal and spatial characteristics of gait during performance of the dynamic gait index in people with and people without balance or vestibular disorders. *Phys Ther.* 2008;88(5):640-651.
5. Murray MP, Drought AB, Kory RC. Walking patterns of normal men. *J Bone Joint Surg Am.* 1964;46:335-360.
6. Murray MP, Kory RC, Sepic SB. Walking patterns of normal women. *Arch Phys Med Rehabil.* 1970;51(11):637-650.
7. Menz HB, Latt MD, Tiedemann A, Mun San Kwan M, Lord SR. Reliability of the GAITRite walkway system for the quantification of temporo-spatial parameters of gait in young and older people. *Gait Posture.* 2004;20(1):20-25.
8. Levinger P, Lai DT, Menz HB, et al. Swing limb mechanics and minimum toe clearance in people with knee osteo-arthritis. *Gait Posture.* 2012;35(2):277-281.
9. Moosabhoy MA, Gard SA. Methodology for determining the sensitivity of swing leg toe clearance and leg length to swing leg joint angles during gait. *Gait Posture.* 2006;24(4):493-501.
10. Saunders JB, Inman VT, Eberhart HD. The major determinants in normal and pathological gait. *J Bone Joint Surg Am.* 1953;35-A(3):543-558.
11. Kerrigan DC, Riley PO, Lelas JL, Della Croce U. Quantification of pelvic rotation as a determinant of gait. *Arch Phys Med Rehabil.* 2001;82(2):217-220.
12. Della Croce U, Riley PO, Lelas JL, Kerrigan DC. A refined view of the determinants of gait. *Gait Posture.* 2001;14(2):79-84.
13. Kerrigan DC, Della Croce U, Marciello M, Riley PO. A refined view of the determinants of gait: significance of heel rise. *Arch Phys Med Rehabil.* 2000;81(8):1077-1080.
14. Lin YC, Gfoehler M, Pandy MG. Quantitative evaluation of the major determinants of human gait. *J Biomech.* 2014;47(6):1324-1331.
15. Orendurff MS, Segal AD, Klute GK, Berge JS, Rohr ES, Kadel NJ. The effect of walking speed on center of mass displacement. *J Rehabil Res Dev.* 2004;41(6A):829-834.

Chapter 3

Normal Gait Kinematics

3.1: DEFINITIONS

Kinematics: A description of movement without concern for the forces causing the movement.

Translational Movement (Linear Displacement): Motion that occurs in one plane (without an axis of rotation). An example includes the curvilinear double sinusoidal center of mass (COM) vertical displacement during walking.

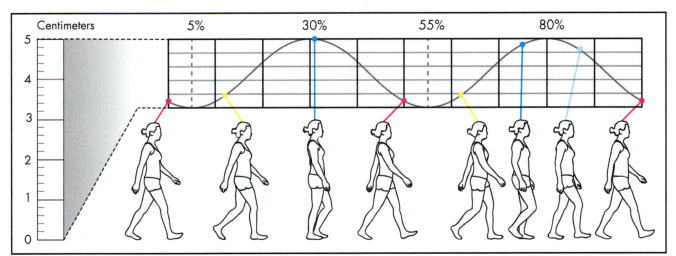

Figure 3-1. Example of a translational movement (COM's vertical displacement). (Adapted from Orendurff MS, Segal AD, Klute GK, Berge JS, Rohr ES, Kadel NJ. The effect of walking speed on center of mass displacement. *J Rehabil Res Dev.* 2004;41[6A]:829-834.)

Adams JM, Cerny K.
Observational Gait Analysis: A Visual Guide (pp 21-58).
© 2018 SLACK Incorporated.

Rotational Movement (Angular Displacement): Motion about an axis of rotation.

An example includes the angular displacement of the tibia about the ankle axis during Mid Stance ankle rocker.

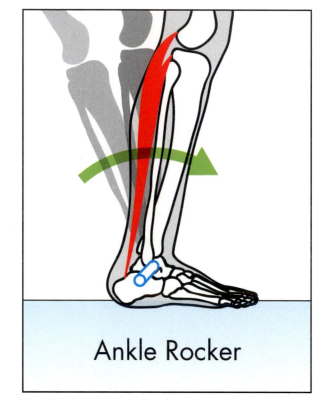

Ankle Rocker

Figure 3-2. An example of a rotational movement (tibia rotation about the ankle axis) during Mid Stance ankle rocker.

3.2: ACQUISITION OF KINEMATIC DATA DURING WALKING

Kinematics Graphs[1]

Typically data collected during an instrumented gait analysis includes kinematics (position and orientation of body segments); foot floor ground reaction forces (using a forceplate); muscle activity (electromyography), preferably using wire electrodes; and temporal-spatial measurements. Most of the kinematic data presented in this chapter were published by Kadaba et al,[1] who used a 5-camera Vicon motion capture system to track the trajectories of reflective markers placed on specific anatomical landmarks. Subjects were asked to walk barefoot, at a comfortable self-selected speed. Sagittal, frontal, and transverse plane kinematics were calculated for 40 individuals (28 males, 12 females), during 3 trials/day, over 3 test days (9 trials/subject). Using a link segment model, joint angles and moments were calculated and normalized for 0% to 100% of the gait cycle (GC).

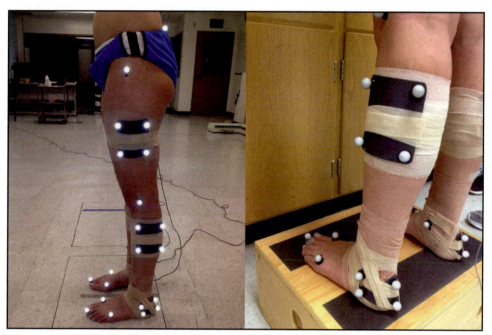

Figure 3-3. Hybrid marker system used with the Vicon Motion Analysis System at the Pathokinesiology Lab of California State University, Long Beach.

3.3: Introduction to Kinematic Joint Graphs Across Phases of the Gait Cycle

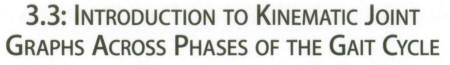

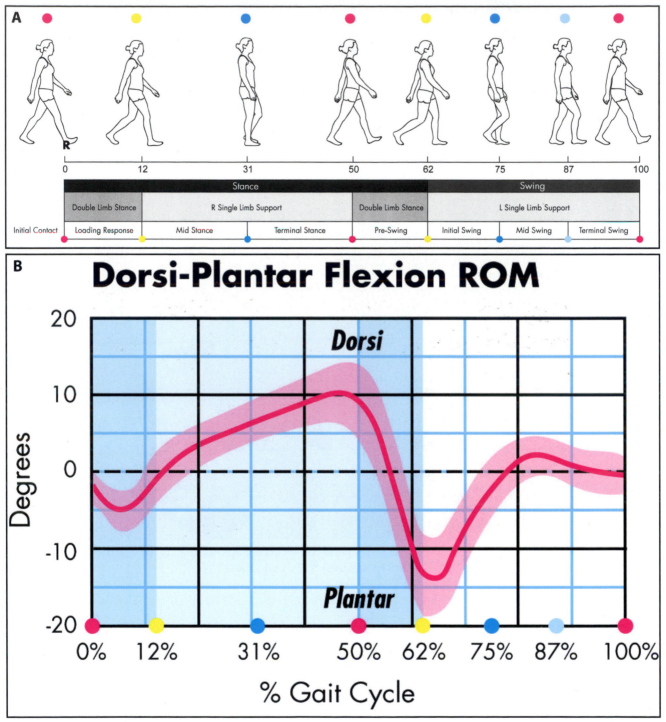

Figure 3-4. (A) Phases of the gait cycle. (B) Ankle kinematic graph. Pink shading represents ± one standard deviation (SD).

Key for Interpreting Graphs

The following key should be used for all the kinematic and kinetic summary graphs. The shading represents periods of double limb stance (DLS), single limb support (SLS), and swing periods, while the colored circles define the individual gait phases.

Shading Key
(Defines Double Limb Stance, Single Limb Support, and Swing)

☐ 0% to 12% GC: Initial Contact and Loading Response
(initial DLS shaded medium blue)

☐ 12% to 50% GC: Mid Stance and Terminal Stance
(SLS shaded light blue)

☐ 50% to 62% GC: Pre-Swing
(terminal DLS shaded medium blue)

☐ 62% to 100% GC: Swing phase (white)

Circle Key
(Defines Phases)

Stance: 0% to 62% GC (Right lower extremity [LE] is the reference limb)

● **Initial Contact (0% to 2% GC)**
The first pink circle marks Initial Contact.

● **Loading Response (2% to 12% GC)**
The first yellow circle marks the end of Loading Response at 12% GC.

● **Mid Stance (12% to 31% GC)**
The turquoise circle marks the end of Mid Stance at 31% GC.

● **Terminal Stance (31% to 50% GC)**
The second pink circle marks the end of Terminal Stance at 50% GC.

● **Pre-Swing (50% to 62% GC)**
The second yellow circle marks the end of Pre-Swing at 62% GC.

Swing: 62% to 100% GC (Right LE is the reference limb)

● **Initial Swing (62% to 75% GC)**
The second turquoise circle marks the end of Initial Swing at 75% GC.

● **Mid Swing (75% to 87% GC)**
The light blue circle marks the end of Mid Swing at 87% GC.

● **Terminal Swing (87% to 100% GC)**
The last pink circle marks the end of Terminal Swing at 100% GC.

Sagittal Kinematic Summary Graphs

Metatarsophalangeal-Hallux Extension (Dorsiflexion) Range of Motion

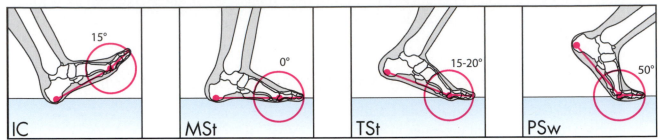

Figure 3-5. Hallux metatarsophalangeal (MTP) range of motion (ROM). (Adapted from Bojsen-Moller F, Lamoreux L. Significance of free-dorsiflexion of the toes in walking. *Acta Orthop Scand.* 1979;50[4]:471-479; Simon J, Doederlein L, McIntosh AS, Metaxiotis D, Bock HG, Wolf SI. The Heidelberg foot measurement method: development, description, and assessment. *Gait Posture.* 2006;23[4]:411-424; Kuni B, Wolf SI, Zeifang F, Thomsen M. Foot kinematics in walking on a level surface and on stairs in patients with hallux rigidus before and after cheilectomy. *J Foot Ankle Res.* 2014;7[1]:13.)

TABLE 3-1	
PHASES	**MOTION**
Initial Contact:	15 degrees extension (DF)
Loading Response:	Flexing to neutral
Mid Stance:	Neutral
Terminal Stance:	15 to 20 degrees extension (DF)
Pre-Swing:	50 degrees extension (DF)
Initial Swing:	Flexing to neutral
Mid Swing:	Neutral
Terminal Swing:	15 degrees extension (DF)
DF: dorsiflexion	

3.4: SAGITTAL PLANE KINEMATICS BY JOINT

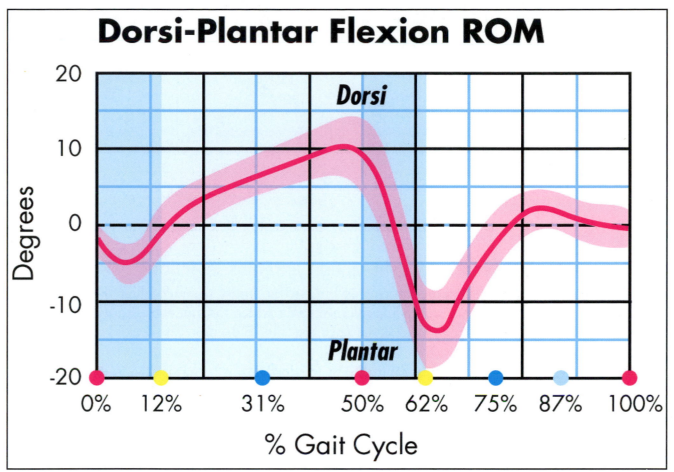

Figure 3-4B. Ankle kinematic graph.

TABLE 3-2	
PHASES	MOTION
Initial Contact:	Neutral
Loading Response:	Plantar flexing to 5 degrees plantar flexion (PF)
Mid Stance:	Dorsiflexing to 5 degrees DF
Terminal Stance:	Dorsiflexing to 10 degrees (DF; roll-off)
Pre-Swing:	Plantar flexing to 15 degrees (PF)
Initial Swing:	Dorsiflexing to 5 degrees (PF)
Mid Swing:	Dorsiflexing to neutral (critical for foot clearance)
Terminal Swing:	Remains dorsiflexed at neutral

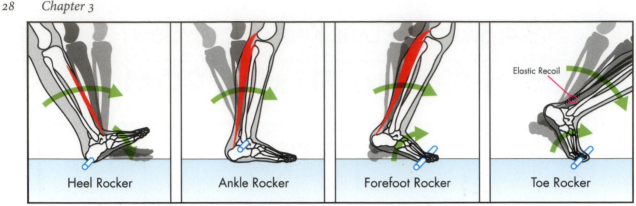

Figure 3-6. Rockers (heel, ankle, forefoot, and toe).

Ankle-Foot Rockers

Perry[2] describes 4 key rockers during stance that contribute to efficient smooth forward progression, minimizing the COM excursion and conserving energy.

Rocker: Description, Phase, Joint Motion, and Muscle Action[2,3]

Heel Rocker (First Rocker): The heel rocker is initiated at Initial Contact when the calcaneus contacts the support surface, and is the fulcrum about which the foot rotates during Loading Response bringing the tibia forward as the knee flexes to 15 degrees. The heel lever causes the ankle to plantar flex 5 degrees.

> **Muscle Action:** PF is eccentrically controlled by the dorsiflexors (anterior tibialis, extensor hallucis longus, and extensor digitorum longus).

Ankle Rocker (Second Rocker): The ankle rocker occurs during Mid Stance when the tibia rotates forward about the talocrural axis resulting in 5 degrees of DF. The tibia progresses over the talus moving the ground reaction force vector anterior to the ankle joint.

> **Muscle Action:** Tibial advancement (DF) is controlled eccentrically by the plantar flexors (primarily soleus and gastrocnemius).

Forefoot Rocker (Third Rocker): The forefoot rocker occurs during Terminal Stance when the heel lifts off the support surface and the mid and hindfoot rotate about the extending metatarsophalangeal (MTP) joints. Ankle DF progresses to 10 degrees as the tibia continues to advance about the ankle axis. Perry's preferred term for this action is *roll-off*, since the plantar flexors eccentrically control DF over the forefoot rocker.[2]

> **Muscle Action:** Eccentric action of the plantar flexors (primarily soleus and gastrocnemius) controls tibial advancement and continued DF.

Toe Rocker (Fourth Rocker): The toe rocker occurs during Pre-Swing when the limb is rapidly unloaded, and weight is transferred to the contralateral limb. The Hallux MTP joint extends to 50 degrees, the ankle plantar flexes to 15 degrees, and the knee flexes to 40 degrees in preparation for swing. Passive elastic recoil of the plantar flexors contributes to knee flexion and forward progression.[2,3]

> **Muscle Action:** Elastic recoil of the Achilles tendon following eccentric action of the soleus and gastrocnemius in the previous phase of Terminal Stance.[2,3] During Pre-Swing passive recoil of the Achilles tendon induces 15 degrees of PF as the limb is rapidly unloaded. Thus, PF arises primarily from stored elastic energy from the stretched Achilles tendon, and is not a result of dynamic muscle activity.[2]

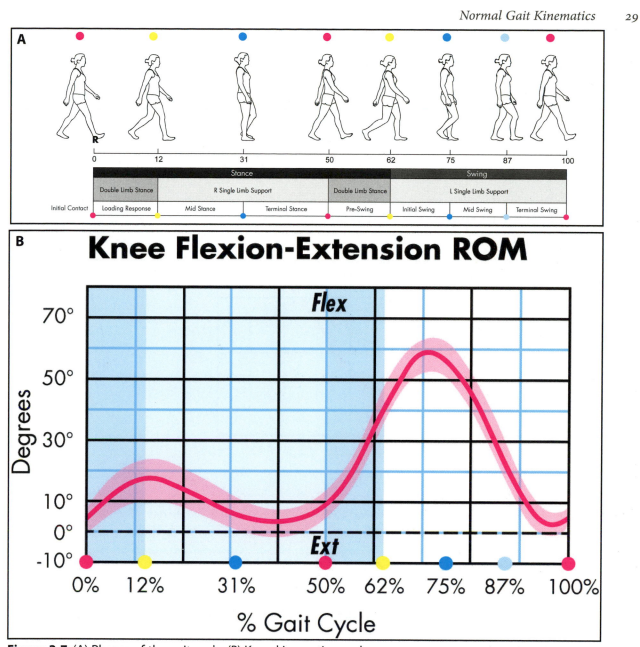

Figure 3-7. (A) Phases of the gait cycle. (B) Knee kinematic graph.

TABLE 3-3	
PHASES	**MOTION**
Initial Contact:	0 ± 5 degrees flexion
Loading Response:	Flexing to 15 degrees
Mid Stance:	Extending
Terminal Stance:	Extending to neutral
Pre-Swing:	Flexing to 40 degrees (critical to achieve peak flexion in Initial Swing)
Initial Swing:	Flexing to 60 degrees (critical for foot clearance)
Mid Swing:	Extending to 25 degrees flexion
Terminal Swing:	Extending to neutral

Thigh vs Hip Kinematics

In order to identify whether the angle/position of the hip joint is due to pelvis or thigh position, the pelvis and thigh are analyzed separately during an observational analysis.[4] The thigh position is referenced to vertical, while true hip position is referenced to the pelvis and is defined as the angle between the pelvis and femur **(Figure 3-8)**.

For example, reference to vertical shows that thigh extension peaks at 15 degrees in Terminal Stance, although the hip joint only reaches approximately 5 degrees because the pelvis is anteriorly tilted.

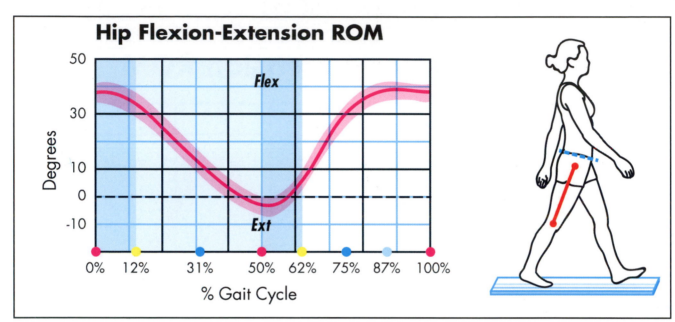

Figure 3-8. Hip kinematic graph (angle referenced to pelvis). The hip joint only reaches ~ 5 degrees of extension.

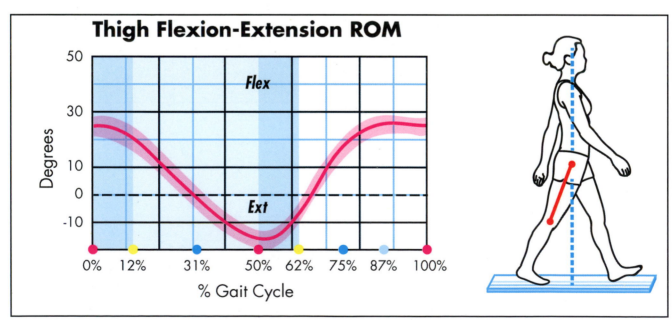

Figure 3-9. Thigh kinematic graph (angle referenced to vertical). The thigh segment reaches ~ 15 degrees of extension.

TABLE 3-4	
PHASES	MOTION (RELATIVE TO VERTICAL)
Initial Contact and Loading Response:	~25 degrees flexion
Mid Stance:	Extending to neutral
Terminal Stance:	Extending to ~15 degrees extension
Pre-Swing:	Flexing toward neutral
Initial Swing:	Flexing to 15 degrees
Mid Swing:	Flexing to 25 degrees
Terminal Swing:	Remaining flexed at 25 degrees

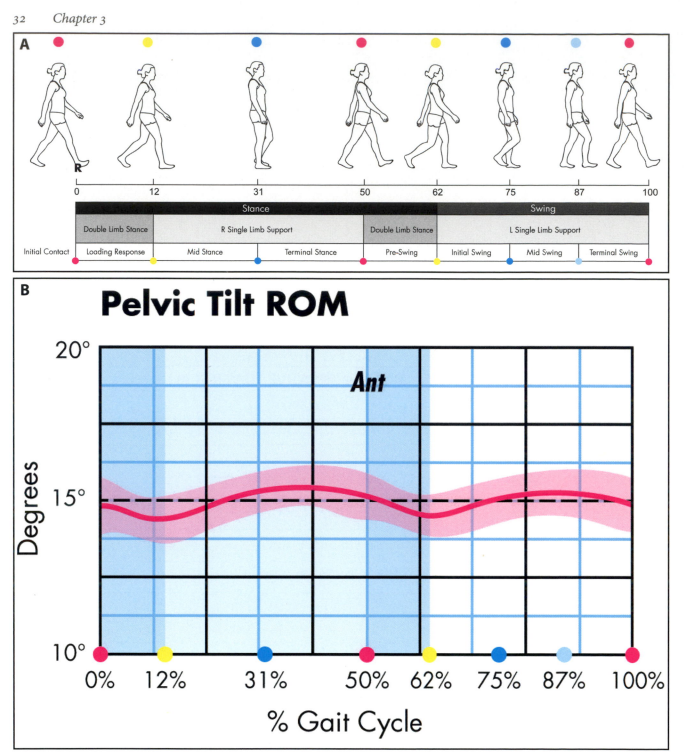

Figure 3-10. (A) Phases of the gait cycle. (B) Pelvic kinematic graph.

Note: During standing, the pelvis is oriented an average of 12 degrees ± 4.5 degrees of tilt anteriorly (angle between the horizontal and a line drawn between the posterior superior iliac spine [PSIS] and anterior superior iliac spine [ASIS]).[5,6] Therefore, pelvic motion during walking is referenced to this position on the kinematic graph. When walking at a comfortable speed, pelvic motion is minimal (2 to 3 degrees), maintaining a posture of approximately 14 to 16 degrees of anterior pelvic tilt (APT) throughout the GC.

TABLE 3-5	
PHASES	MOTION (RELATIVE TO VERTICAL)
Initial Contact:	~ 15 degrees of APT
Loading Response:	Tilting posteriorly (relative) to ~ 14 degrees of APT
Mid Stance:	Tilting anteriorly to 15 degrees
Terminal Stance:	Peak at 16 degrees of APT then begins tilting posteriorly (relative) at 40% GC
Pre-Swing:	Continues tilting posteriorly (relative) to ~ 14 degrees of APT
Initial Swing:	Tilting anteriorly
Mid Swing:	Continues tilting anteriorly
Terminal Swing:	Tilting posteriorly to 15 degrees of APT

3.5: SAGITTAL KINEMATIC SUMMARY ACROSS JOINTS FOR EACH PHASE OF THE GAIT CYCLE

Initial Contact

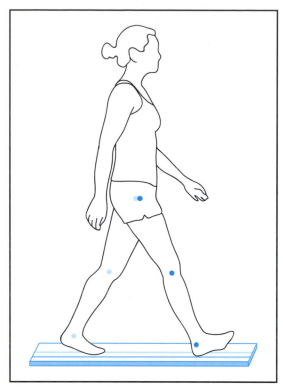

Figure 3-11. Initial Contact (0% to 2% GC).

TABLE 3-6. SAGITTAL PLANE KINEMATICS AT INITIAL CONTACT	
JOINT/SEGMENT	**DEGREES/POSITION**
Ankle	0 degrees neutral
Knee	0 ± 5 degrees
Thigh **(referenced to vertical)**	25 degrees flexion
Pelvis **(referenced to horizontal)**	15 degrees anterior tilt
Trunk	0 degrees neutral

CRITICAL EVENT
HEEL CONTACT
Heel contact initiates the heel rocker by creating an external PF moment at the ankle initiating PF.

Loading Response

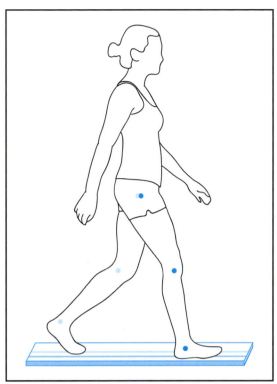

Figure 3-12. Loading Response (2% to 12% GC).

TABLE 3-7. SAGITTAL PLANE KINEMATICS DURING LOADING RESPONSE	
JOINT/SEGMENT	**DEGREES/POSITION**
Ankle	5 degrees PF
Knee	15 degrees flexion
Thigh **(referenced to vertical)**	25 degrees flexion
Pelvis **(referenced to horizontal)**	~ 14 degrees anterior tilt
Trunk	0 degrees neutral

CRITICAL EVENTS
CONTROLLED KNEE FLEXION AND PF (HEEL ROCKER) WITH HIP STABILIZATION DURING WEIGHT TRANSFER
Following heel contact at Initial Contact, the heel rocker causes the forefoot to descend to the floor around the calcaneus/floor axis, and the heel lever causes 5 degrees of PF. As the tibia simultaneously advances forward, no further ankle PF occurs, and tibial forward rotation causes the knee to flex 15 degrees. The thigh is stable as it begins to extend with the trunk upright. Knee flexion and PF decelerate body weight to absorb shock.

Mid Stance

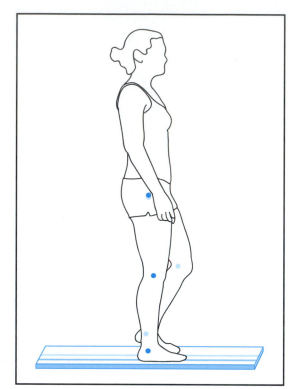

Figure 3-13. Mid Stance (12% to 31% GC).

TABLE 3-8. SAGITTAL PLANE KINEMATICS DURING MID STANCE	
JOINT/SEGMENT	**DEGREES/POSITION**
Ankle	5 degrees DF
Knee	0 degrees neutral
Thigh (referenced to vertical)	0 degrees neutral
Pelvis (referenced to horizontal)	15 degrees anterior tilt
Trunk	0 degrees neutral

CRITICAL EVENT
CONTROLLED ANKLE DF WITH FOOT FLAT (ANKLE ROCKER)
The tibia rotates forward at the ankle (ankle rocker) over the plantigrade foot into 5 degrees of DF. The ground reaction force vector (GRFV) advances from posterior to anterior at the ankle joint.

...

Terminal Stance

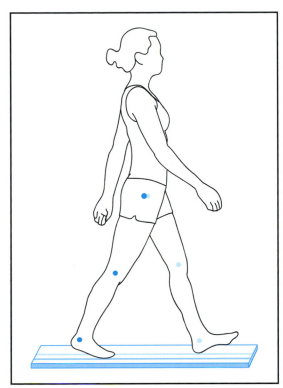

Figure 3-14. Terminal Stance (31% to 50% GC).

TABLE 3-9. SAGITTAL PLANE KINEMATICS DURING TERMINAL STANCE	
JOINT/SEGMENT	**DEGREES/POSITION**
Ankle	10 degrees DF
Knee	0 degrees neutral
Thigh (referenced to vertical)	15 degrees extension
Pelvis (referenced to horizontal)	~ 16 degrees anterior tilt
Trunk	0 degrees neutral

CRITICAL EVENTS
THIGH EXTENSION WITH CONTROLLED ANKLE DF AND HEEL RISE
The tibia continues to advance forward into 10 degrees of DF as the thigh extends 15 degrees from vertical, creating contralateral step length. The heel rises, extending (dorsiflexing) the MTP joints (forefoot rocker), as the GRFV advances forward. Perry's preferred term for this action is *roll-off*

Pre-Swing

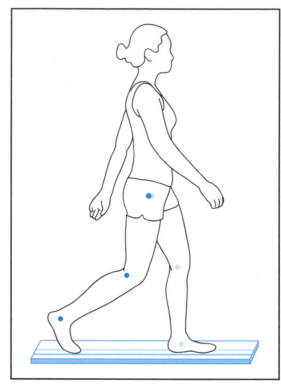

Figure 3-15. Pre-Swing (50% to 62% GC).

TABLE 3-10. SAGITTAL PLANE KINEMATICS DURING PRE-SWING	
JOINT/SEGMENT	DEGREES/POSITION
Ankle	15 degrees PF
Knee	40 degrees flexion
Thigh **(referenced to vertical)**	Neutral
Pelvis **(referenced to horizontal)**	~15 degrees anterior tilt
Trunk	0 degrees neutral

CRITICAL EVENTS
THIGH FLEXION TO NEUTRAL, PASSIVE KNEE FLEXION TO 40 DEGREES, AND ANKLE PF OF 15 DEGREES DURING LIMB UNLOADING
Momentum from thigh flexion and elastic recoil from the plantar flexors[3] cause the knee to passively flex to 40 degrees, as the GRFV advances onto the phalanges (toe rocker) in preparation for swing. Knee flexion of 40 degrees in this phase (Pre-Swing) is critical for toe clearance in Initial Swing when 60 degrees of knee flexion is expected.

Initial Swing

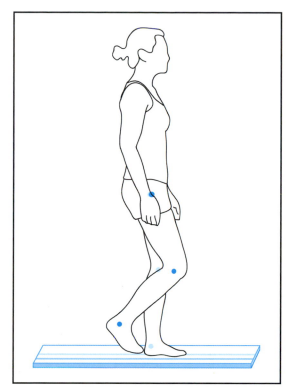

Figure 3-16. Initial Swing (62% to 75% GC).

TABLE 3-11. SAGITTAL PLANE KINEMATICS DURING INITIAL SWING	
JOINT/SEGMENT	**DEGREES/POSITION**
Ankle	5 degrees PF
Knee	60 degrees flexion
Thigh **(referenced to vertical)**	15 degrees flexion
Pelvis **(referenced to horizontal)**	~ 15 degrees anterior tilt
Trunk	0 degrees neutral

CRITICAL EVENTS
THIGH FLEXION TO 15 DEGREES AND KNEE FLEXION TO 60 DEGREES
Knee flexion of 60 degrees clears the plantar flexed foot from the floor, while thigh flexion advances the limb forward.

Mid Swing

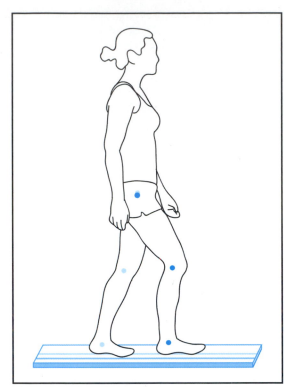

Figure 3-17. Mid Swing (75% to 87% GC).

TABLE 3-12. SAGITTAL PLANE KINEMATICS DURING MID SWING	
JOINT/SEGMENT	DEGREES/POSITION
Ankle	0 degrees neutral
Knee	25 degrees flexion
Thigh (referenced to vertical)	25 degrees flexion
Pelvis (referenced to horizontal)	15 degrees anterior tilt
Trunk	0 degrees neutral

CRITICAL EVENTS
ANKLE DF TO NEUTRAL, THIGH FLEXION, AND KNEE EXTENSION
Continued thigh flexion and beginning knee extension advance the limb forward for step length. Ankle DF to neutral clears the toes from the floor as the knee extends.

Terminal Swing

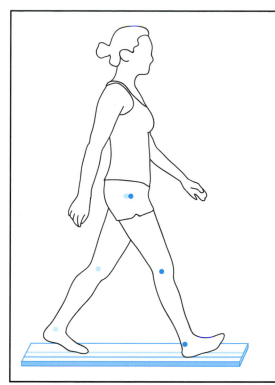

Figure 3-18. Terminal Swing (87% to 100% GC).

TABLE 3-13. SAGITTAL PLANE KINEMATICS DURING TERMINAL SWING	
JOINT/SEGMENT	DEGREES/POSITION
Ankle	0 degrees neutral
Knee	0 degrees neutral
Thigh **(referenced to vertical)**	25 degrees flexion
Pelvis **(referenced to horizontal)**	15 degrees anterior tilt
Trunk	0 degrees neutral

CRITICAL EVENT
KNEE EXTENSION TO NEUTRAL
Knee extension advances the limb, creates step length, and positions the heel for Initial Contact (heel rocker).

3.6: Minimal Foot/Toe Clearance in Swing: Key Kinematic Events

Foot/toe clearance is dependent on the coordinated motions of the lower extremities and pelvis of both the swing and stance limbs. For safe, unimpeded, forward progression, toe clearance is critical. *Minimum toe clearance* (MTC) is defined as the minimal distance between the toes and the contact surface during swing, and is relatively small (1 to 2 cm).[7,8] With minimal clearance there is a small margin of error to prevent toe contact and possible tripping. During Initial Swing, toe clearance is most sensitive to knee flexion (normally 60 degrees).[7]

Initial Swing Critical Event for Toe/Foot Clearance: Knee Flexion to 60 Degrees

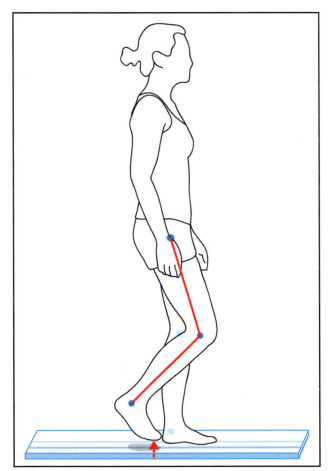

Figure 3-19. Initial Swing knee flexion (60 degrees) for minimal toe clearance.

Mid Swing Critical Event for Toe/Foot Clearance: Dorsiflexion to Neutral

In contrast, toe clearance during Mid Swing is most sensitive to ankle DF. This is when the ankle normally reaches neutral, while the knee is extending (relatively lengthening the limb) as the thigh moves forward. Clinically this is an important distinction since toe drag during Initial Swing is primarily related to inadequate knee flexion, while toe drag during Mid Swing is related to inadequate DF.

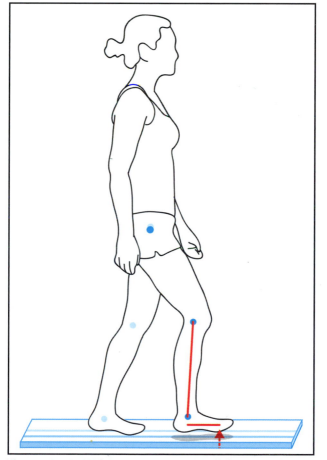

Figure 3-20. Mid Swing DF to neutral for minimal toe clearance.

3.7: Frontal Plane Kinematic Summary Graphs

Calcaneal Motion Summary

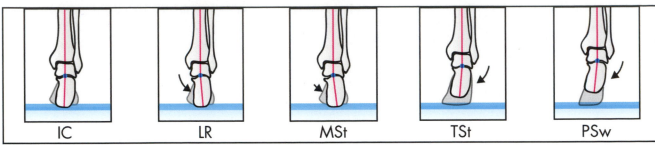

Figure 3-21. Calcaneal inversion/eversion kinematics.

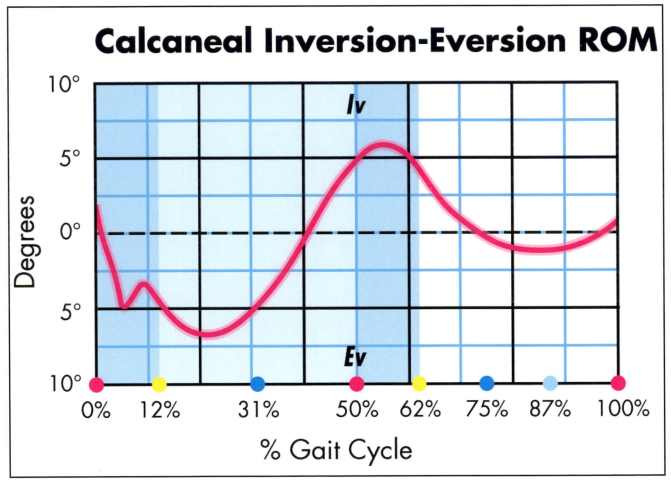

Figure 3-22. Calcaneal inversion/eversion kinematics graph. (Adapted from Wright DG, Desai SM, Henderson WH. Action of the subtalar and ankle joint complex during the stance phase of walking. *J Bone Joint Surg Am.* 1964;46:361-382.)

TABLE 3-14. FRONTAL PLANE FOOT KINEMATICS SUMMARY			
PHASE	**CALCANEUS**	**SUBTALAR MOTION**	**TRANSVERSE TARSAL FUNCTION**
Initial Contact	2 degrees inversion (Iv)	Supinated	Loading
Loading Response	Everting to 5 degrees eversion (Ev)	Pronating	Unlocking (increased flexibility)
Early Mid Stance	Peak eversion (Ev) (7 degrees)	Pronating	Unlocked
Late Mid Stance	Inverting to 5 degrees Ev	Supinating	Locking (motion suppression)
Terminal Stance	Inverting to 5 degrees inversion (Iv)	Supinating	Locked (motion suppression)
Pre-Swing	6 degrees Iv	Supinated	Unloading
Total Motion:		7 degrees eversion to 6 degrees inversion (13 degrees)	

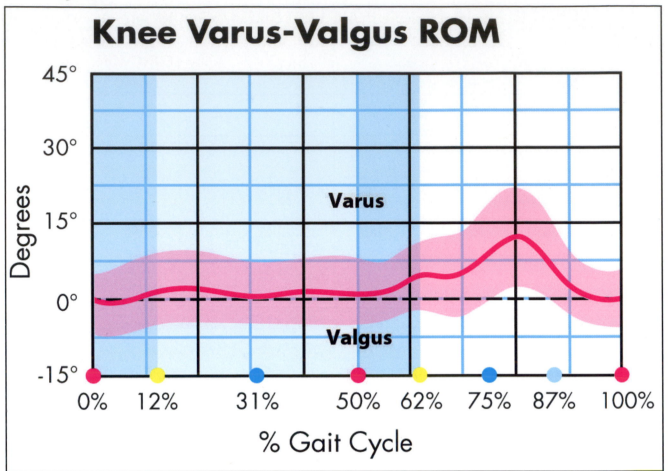

Figure 3-23. Knee varus/valgus kinematic graph. Note: frontal plane knee motion is minimal during stance (2 to 3 degrees).

TABLE 3-15	
PHASES	MOTION
Initial Contact and Loading Response:	Minimal valgus
Mid Stance:	Minimal varus
Terminal Stance:	Minimal varus
Pre-Swing:	Increasing varus
Initial Swing:	Increasing varus
Mid Swing:	Peak varus (12 degrees)
Terminal Swing:	Decreasing varus
Total Motion:	Slight valgus to 12 degrees varus

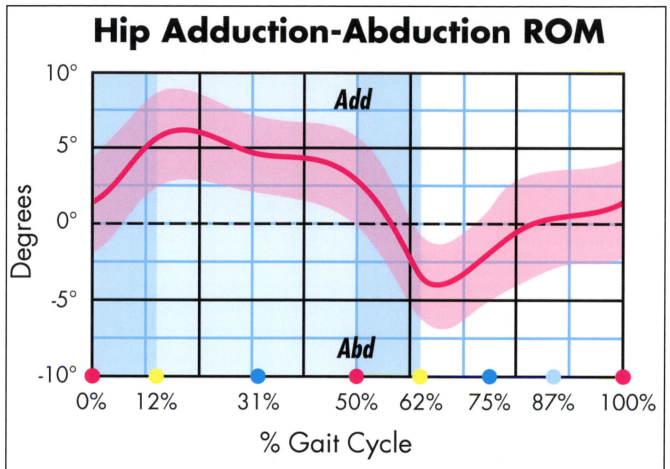

Figure 3-24. Hip adduction/abduction kinematic graph.

TABLE 3-16	
PHASES	MOTION
Initial Contact and Loading Response:	Adducted
Mid Stance:	Peak adduction (~5 degrees; due to left pelvic drop)
Terminal Stance:	Abducting toward neutral
Pre-Swing:	Neutral
Initial Swing:	Peak Abduction (~5 degrees; due to left pelvic elevation to neutral)
Mid Swing and Terminal Swing:	Adducting
Total Motion:	Neutral to 5 degrees

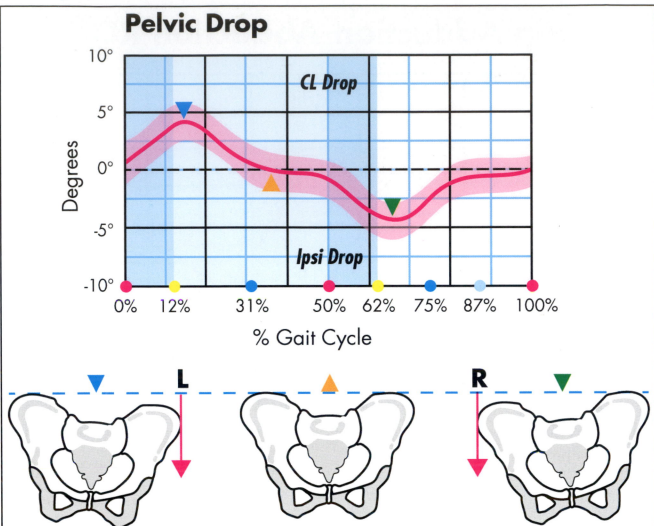

Figure 3-25. Pelvic frontal plane kinematic graph.

TABLE 3-17	
PHASES	MOTION
Initial Contact and Loading Response:	Left (CL) side of pelvis dropping from neutral
Mid Stance:	Peak left drop (~5 degrees) in early Mid Stance; then left side begins elevating toward neutral
Terminal Stance:	Left side elevating to neutral
Pre-Swing:	Right (Ipsi) side of pelvis dropping from neutral
Initial Swing:	Peak right (Ipsi) drop (~5 degrees) in early Initial Swing; then right side begins elevating toward neutral
Mid Swing and Terminal Swing:	Right side elevating to neutral
Total Motion:	Neutral to 5 degree drop on each side

3.8: TRANSVERSE PLANE KINEMATIC SUMMARY GRAPHS

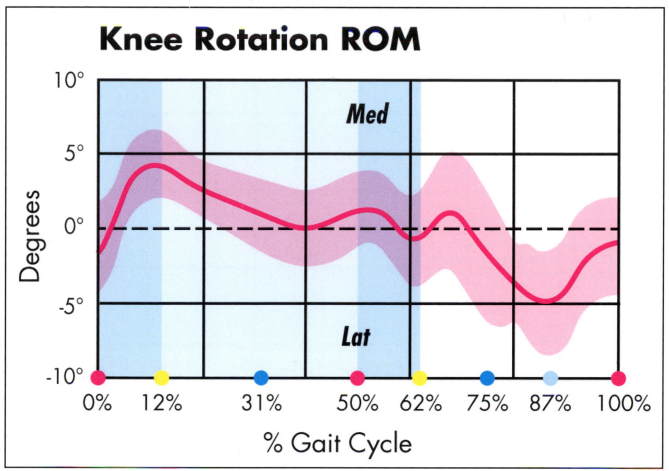

Figure 3-26. Knee rotation (medial/lateral) kinematic graph.

TABLE 3-18	
PHASES	MOTION
Initial Contact:	Laterally rotated (slight)
Loading Response:	Medially rotating to peak (~ 5 degrees)
Mid Stance:	Laterally rotating
Terminal Stance:	Continues laterally rotating to neutral
Pre-Swing:	Neutral
Initial Swing:	Neutral
Mid Swing:	Laterally rotating to 5 degrees of lateral rotation
Terminal Swing:	Medially rotating back toward neutral
Total Motion:	5 degrees medial rotation to 5 degrees lateral

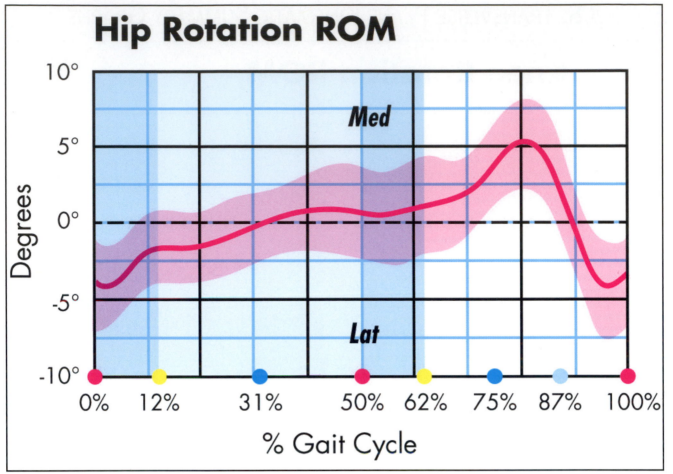

Figure 3-27. Hip rotation (medial/lateral) kinematic graph.

TABLE 3-19	
PHASES	HIP: ROTATION MOTION GRAPH
Initial Contact:	Peak lateral rotation (5 degrees)
Loading Response:	Medially rotating
Mid Stance:	Medially rotating to neutral
Terminal Stance:	Medially rotating
Pre-Swing:	Medially rotating
Initial Swing:	Medially rotating
Mid Swing:	Medially rotated to peak (5 degrees of medial rotation)
Terminal Swing:	Laterally rotating to peak (5 degrees of lateral rotation)
Total Motion:	10 degrees

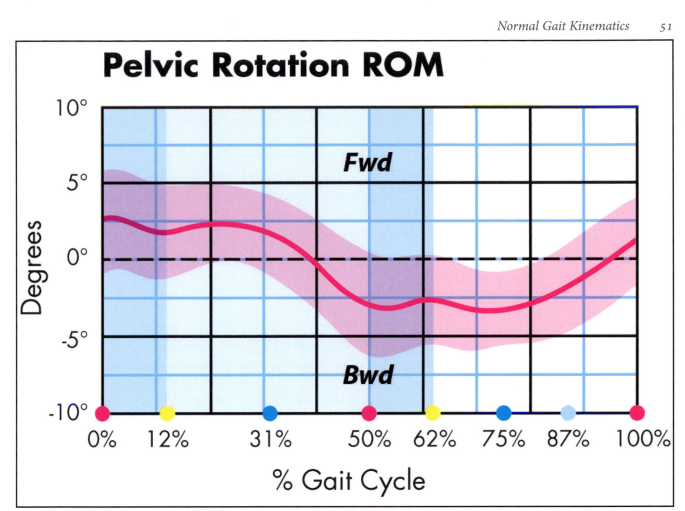

Figure 3-28. Pelvic forward/backward rotation kinematic graph.

TABLE 3-20	
PHASES	MOTION
Initial Contact:	Peak forward rotation (~3 to 5 degrees)
Loading Response:	Peak forward rotation (~3 to 5 degrees)
Mid Stance:	Remains rotated forward
Terminal Stance:	Rotating backward
Pre-Swing:	Peak backward rotation (~3 to 5 degrees)
Initial Swing:	Peak backward rotation (~3 to 5 degrees)
Mid Swing:	Rotating forward (~3 to 5 degrees)
Terminal Swing:	Rotating forward (~3 to 5 degrees)
Total Motion:	Highly variable; approximately 3 to 5 degrees forward and 3 to 5 degrees backward rotation

Reciprocal Arm Swing

Arm swing is an integral component of normal gait and has both active and passive components. Minimal muscle activation (electromyograph < 5% maximum voluntary isometric contraction) of the shoulder flexor and extensor muscles, including both shortening and lengthening contractions, initiates and controls arm excursion.[9] The shoulder's total excursion averages (flexion and extension) 20 to 26 degrees.[10] Reciprocal arm swing decreases the vertical ground reaction moments, minimizing energy expenditure.[10,11] As shown in Figure 3-29, when the right shoulder is maximally flexed at the end of Terminal Stance and beginning of Pre-Swing, the pelvis is maximally rotated backward. These motions counterbalance one another, limiting trunk angular momentum. As walking speed increases, both the total arc of shoulder motion and the arc of pelvic rotation increase.[2]

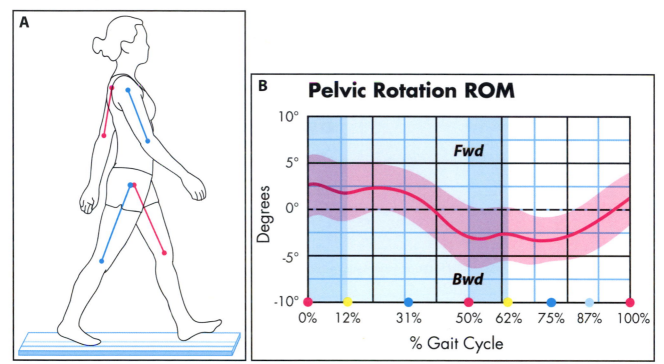

Figure 3-29. (A) Reciprocal arm swing. (B) Pelvic forward/backward rotation kinematic graph.

3.9: FRONTAL PLANE KINEMATICS BY PHASE

Loading Response (2% to 12% Gait Cycle)

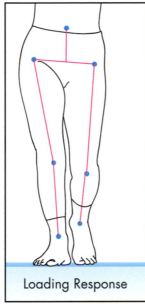

Figure 3-30. Frontal plane kinematics during Loading Response (anterior view for pelvis, thigh, and knee).

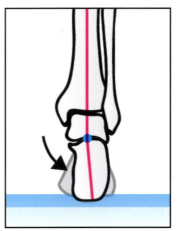

Figure 3-31. Frontal plane kinematics during Loading Response (posterior view for calcaneus).

TABLE 3-21. FRONTAL PLANE KINEMATICS DURING LOADING RESPONSE	
JOINT/SEGMENT	**DEGREES/POSITION**
***Calcaneus* (referenced to tibia)**	Everting
Knee	Minimal valgus (abduction)
Hip	5 degrees adduction
***Pelvis* (referenced to horizontal)**	Contralateral drop from neutral
Trunk	Erect

CRITICAL EVENT
CALCANEAL EVERSION COUPLED WITH MEDIAL TIBIAL ROTATION DURING WEIGHT TRANSFER
Calcaneal eversion unlocks the foot and increases its flexibility, while body weight is being transferred to the stance limb.

Mid Stance (12% to 31% Gait Cycle)

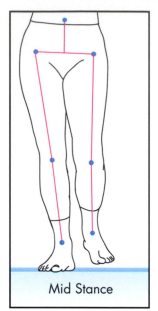

Mid Stance

Figure 3-32. Anterior view for frontal plane kinematics during Mid Stance.

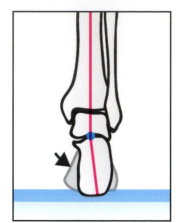

Figure 3-33. Posterior calcaneal view.

TABLE 3-22. FRONTAL PLANE KINEMATICS DURING MID STANCE	
JOINT/SEGMENT	**DEGREES/POSITION**
Calcaneus (referenced to tibia)	Continues everting to peak of 7 degrees Ev before beginning relative inversion
Knee	Minimal adduction (distal tibia; varus)
Hip	Remains minimally adducted
Pelvis (referenced to horizontal)	Less contralateral drop
Trunk	Erect

CRITICAL EVENT
MINIMAL CONTRALATERAL PELVIC DROP
Minimal CL pelvic drop prevents lengthening of the swing limb, enabling toe clearance.

Terminal Stance (31% to 50% Gait Cycle)

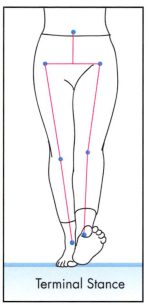

Figure 3-34. Anterior view frontal plane kinematics during Terminal Stance.

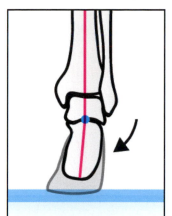

Figure 3-35. Posterior calcaneal view.

TABLE 3-23. FRONTAL PLANE KINEMATICS DURING TERMINAL STANCE	
JOINT/SEGMENT	DEGREES/POSITION
Calcaneus *(referenced to tibia)*	Inverting to 5 degrees inversion
Knee	Minimal adduction (varus)
Hip *(referenced to tibia)*	Less adduction
Pelvis *(referenced to horizontal)*	Neutral
Trunk	Erect

CRITICAL EVENTS
CALCANEAL INVERSION COUPLED WITH LATERAL TIBIAL ROTATION AND PELVIC ROTATION
Calcaneal inversion locks the midfoot, suppresses motion, and provides stability for heel rise and forward propulsion. Backward pelvic rotation during terminal stance with contralateral forward rotation in terminal swing contributes to step length.

3.10: KINEMATIC SUMMARY OF THE KNEE AND FOOT

TABLE 3-24. KINEMATIC SUMMARY OF THE KNEE AND FOOT						
PHASE	**KNEE**	**TIBIA ON FEMUR**	**CALCANEUS**	**SUBTALAR MOTION**	**MIDFOOT FUNCTION**	**FOREFOOT**
Initial Contact	Extended	Laterally rotated	2 degrees inverted	Supinated	Locked	Adducted
Loading Response	Flexing	Medially rotating	Everting to 5 degrees Ev	Pronating	Unlocking (increased flexibility) Absorbing shock	Abducting
Early Mid Stance	Extending	Laterally rotating	Everting to 7 degrees Ev	Pronating	Unlocking	Abducting
Late Mid Stance	Extending	Laterally rotated	Inverting to 5 degrees Ev	Supinating	Locking	Adducting
Terminal Stance	Extended	Laterally rotated	Inverting to 5 degrees Iv	Supinated	Locked (motion suppression)	Adducted
Pre-Swing	Flexing	Medially rotating	6 degrees Iv	Supinated	Unloading	Adducted

3.11: KINEMATIC SUMMARY OF THE LOWER EXTREMITY

Motion	IC	LR	MSt	TSt	PSw	ISw	MSw	TSw
H-MTP	15° X	Flexing	Neutral	15°-20° X	50° X	Flexing	0°	15° X
STJ	2° IV	EV to 5°	EV to 7°	IV to 5° IV	5° IV	IV to 6° IV	Everting	2° IV
Ankle	0°	5° PF	5° DF	10° DF	15° PF	DF to 5° PF	DF to 0°	0°
Knee F/X	0° ± 5°	15°	0°	0°	40°	60°	25°	0°
Knee Rot	Laterally Rotated	M Rotating to 5°	Laterally Rotating	Neutral	Neutral	Neutral	L Rotating to 5°	M Rotating to Neutral
Thigh F/X	25°	25°	0°	15° X	Flexing	15° F	25° F	25°
Hip Rot	LR 5°	Medially Rotating	Medially Rotating	Medially Rotating	Medially Rotating	Medially Rotating	MR 5°	L Rotating to 5°
Hip Ad/Ab	Adducted	Adducted to 6°	Abducting	Abducting	Neutral	Abducted to 5°	Adducting	Adducted
Pelvic Drop	Neutral	CL Dropping	5° CL Drop	Elevating	Neutral	Ipsi Dropping	5° Ipsi Drop	Neutral
Pelvic Rot	≈5° FW	≈5° FW	Rotating BW	BW 5°	BW 5°	Rotating FW	Rotating FW	≈5° FW
Pelvic Tilt	15° AT	14° AT	15° AT	16° AT	14° AT	15° AT	15° AT	15° AT
Trunk	Neutral	Neutral	Neutral	Neutral	Neutral	Neutral	Neutral	Neutral

Figure 3-36. Kinematic summary of the lower extremity.

Figures 3-4, 3-7, 3-8, 3-9, 3-10, 3-23, 3-24, 3-25, 3-26, 3-27, 3-28, and 3-29 are adapted from Kadaba MP, Ramakrishnan HK, Wootten ME. Measurement of lower extremity kinematics during level walking. *J Orthop Res.* 1990;8(3):383-392

3.12: REFERENCES

1. Kadaba MP, Ramakrishnan HK, Wootten ME. Measurement of lower extremity kinematics during level walking. *J Orthop Res.* 1990;8(3):383-392.
2. Perry J, Burnfield JM. *Gait Analysis: Normal & Pathological Gait.* 2nd ed. Thorofare, NJ: SLACK Incorporated; 2010.
3. Fukunaga T, Kubo K, Kawakami Y, Fukashiro S, Kanehisa H, Maganaris CN. In vivo behaviour of human muscle tendon during walking. *Proc Biol Sci.* 2001;268(1464):229-233.
4. Pathokinesiology Service and the Department of Physical Therapy. *Observational Gait Analysis.* 4th ed. Rancho Los Amigos National Rehabilitaton Center, Downey, CA: Los Amigos Research and Educational Institute Inc; 2001.
5. Crowell RD, Cummings GS, Walker JR, Tillman LJ. Intratester and intertester reliability and validity of measures of innominate bone inclination. *J Orthop Sports Phys Ther.* 1994;20(2):88-97.
6. Levine D, Whittle MW. The effects of pelvic movement on lumbar lordosis in the standing position. *J Orthop Sports Phys Ther.* 1996;24(3):130-135.
7. Moosabhoy MA, Gard SA. Methodology for determining the sensitivity of swing leg toe clearance and leg length to swing leg joint angles during gait. *Gait Posture.* 2006;24(4):493-501.
8. Levinger P, Lai DT, Menz HB, et al. Swing limb mechanics and minimum toe clearance in people with knee osteoarthritis. *Gait Posture.* 2012;35(2):277-281.
9. Kuhtz-Buschbeck JP, Jing B. Activity of upper limb muscles during human walking. *J Electromyogr Kinesiol.* 2012;22(2):199-206.
10. Plate A, Sedunko D, Pelykh O, Schlick C, Ilmberger JR, Botzel K. Normative data for arm swing asymmetry: how (a)symmetrical are we? *Gait Posture.* 2015;41(1):13-18.
11. Collins SH, Adamczyk PG, Kuo AD. Dynamic arm swinging in human walking. *Proc Biol Sci.* 2009;276(1673):3679-3688.

Please see videos on the accompanying website at

www.healio.com/books/oga

Chapter 4

Normal Gait Kinetics

4.1: Definitions

Kinetics: The study of forces and their effect on motion.

Force: The "push or pull" of one object on another, measured in Newtons (N). A Newton is the force required to accelerate 1 kg to 1 m/sec^2

Newton's Third Law (Law of Action-Reaction): When a person is standing on the floor, the body exerts a force on the floor while the floor exerts a force "equal in magnitude but opposite in direction" on the body. This force is referred to as the **ground reaction force (GRF)**. The 3 components of the GRF, each representing a different orthogonal direction (vertical, anterior/posterior [A/P], and medio/lateral [M/L]), are typically measured by a force plate embedded in the walking surface.

The GRFs are represented by a vector **(ground reaction force vector [GRFV])**, which is the result of adding the vertical force and shear forces. The sagittal plane GRFV is the addition of the vertical and A/P forces, while the frontal plane vector is composed of the vertical and M/L forces. For example in **Figure 4-1**, the red sagittal plane GRFV of the walking figure is the resultant vector of the vertical (blue) and anterior/posterior (green) GRFs.

The GRFV displayed in the frontal plane **(Figure 4-2)** is the resultant vector of the vertical (blue) and M/L (green) GRFs. The location of the GRFV, when superimposed on a walking figure, can help visualize the external moments created at the lower limb joints. The origin of the GRFV is a single point referred to as the center of pressure (COP), and represents the location of net moments occurring within the base of support (BOS).

Adams JM, Cerny K.
Observational Gait Analysis: A Visual Guide (pp 59-93).
© 2018 SLACK Incorporated.

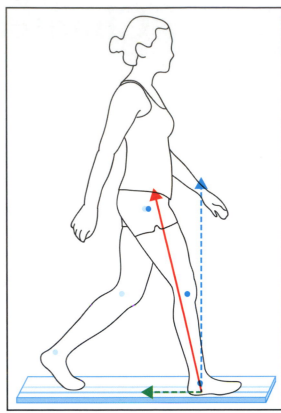

Figure 4-1. Sagittal plane GRFV in red, vertical component in blue, and A/P (fore-aft) component in green.

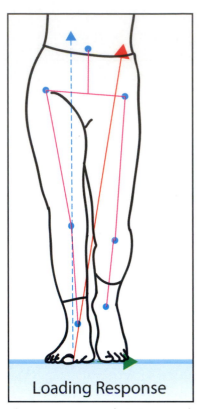

Loading Response

Figure 4-2. Frontal GRFV in red, vertical component in blue, and M/L component in green.

Determination of Joint Moments

Link Segment Model Using Inverse Dynamics

In the lab environment, joint moments are calculated using equations where the body is considered a series of segments linked together (eg, thigh, leg, foot). This analysis requires anthropometric characteristics from each subject (the segment's mass, the segment's center of mass location, the joint centers, and the segment's inertial properties). Also required are precise kinematics (position and orientation of the segments in space and the accelerations of the segment's mass) captured by cameras with the force plates measuring the force of the foot on the support surface. Through a process called *inverse dynamics,* external moments are calculated and internal moments defined and designated by the predominant muscle groups that are presumed active. However, internal moments may also be caused by series elastic elements (eg, ligaments, tendons, joint capsules) without muscle action. Only with intramuscular electromyography (EMG) recordings can one be certain that specific muscles are active, and hence contributing to the force component.

When reading the literature the reader must determine whether internal or external moments are described to interpret the results correctly. In this text, we consistently refer to external moments because we visually interpret joint demand using the position of the limbs relative to the GRFV.

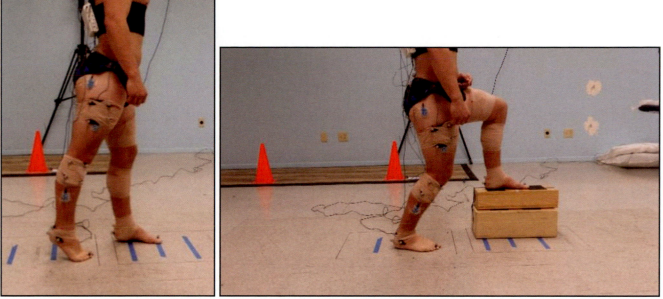

Figure 4-3. Subject is instrumented for joint kinematics and kinetics.

Terminology for Defining External Moments

The *external moment* reflects the effects of gravity and acceleration on the mass of the limb segments.

TABLE 4-1. EXTERNAL MOMENT TERMINOLOGY			
JOINT	**SAGITTAL PLANE**	**FRONTAL PLANE**	**TRANSVERSE PLANE**
Hip	Flexion/extension	Abduction/adduction	M/L rotation
Knee	Flexion/extension	Varus/valgus	M/L rotation
Ankle (subtalar)	PF/DF	Inversion (adduction)/ eversion (abduction)	M/L rotation
PF: plantar flexion; DF: dorsiflexion			

Power

Joint power, or the rate of doing work, is the product of the joint moment multiplied by the joint's angular velocity. Power generation is depicted as positive and is usually associated with concentric contractions, while power absorption is depicted as negative and is associated with eccentric contractions. Internal moments and powers are defined by the angular motion occurring. This has led some to assume that the corresponding flexor and extensor muscles are causing the moments and powers. However, internal joint moments and powers derived from inverse dynamics do not reveal the source of the forces producing the moments and powers. Internal moments may also be caused by passive forces (eg, ligaments, tendon, joint capsules, muscle fascicles, bone). When elastic elements are stretched they store energy by absorbing power and then return the elastic energy by recoil, generating power. Only with intramuscular electromyography (EMG) recordings can one be certain that specific muscles are active and hence, contributing to the joint forces. Even with EMG activity, the magnitude of the active muscle component contributing to force production is impossible to fully determine.

Although the exact contribution of passive structures vs active muscle contraction in power production is difficult to determine, the evidence suggests that the connective tissues contribution is significant in normal walking.

Examples

1. Stretch of the hip flexors during Terminal Stance, when hip flexor muscles are inactive, stores energy that is returned in Pre- and Initial Swing.[1]

2. Stretch of the plantar flexor muscles in Mid and Terminal Stance stores energy that is returned in Pre-Swing to plantar flex the ankle.

Fukunaga et al,[2] using ultrasound images of muscle fascicles and tendon, determined that the medial gastrocnemius muscle exhibited "near isometric behavior" (muscle fascicles maintained a near constant length) in Mid and Terminal Stance when the muscle was active (surface EMG) during treadmill walking. At the same time, he found the Achilles tendon and muscle aponeurosis lengthened placing them on stretch. Then, during Pre-Swing, the muscle shortened, but the gastrocnemius (G) muscle was silent (EMG). He concluded that the Achilles tendon and aponeurosis recoiled causing the muscle to shorten passively. The rapid plantar flexor shortening implies a peak in PF power generation that was primarily due to the passive elastic elements.

4.2: Visualizing the Ground Reaction Force Vector to Determine External Moments

Sagittal Plane

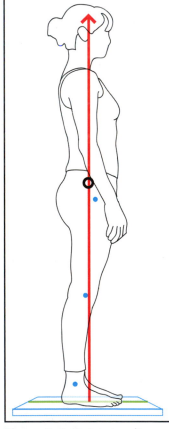

Figure 4-4. Quiet standing sagittal plane with GRFV visualization.

TABLE 4-2. SAGITTAL PLANE GROUND REACTION FORCE VECTOR VISUALIZATION
VISUALIZING THE EXTERNAL MOMENT IN THE SAGITTAL PLANE IN STANDING
GRFV reflects the resultant vertical and fore/aft forces the floor imposes on the body (red line). The magnitude of the GRFV in standing is equal to the mass (kg) times acceleration (gravity = 9.8 m/sec^2) and is expressed in Newtons (N). Because there is minimal motion, the GRFV passes through the body's COM.
COM FOR THE BODY: BLACK CIRCLE
AOR for the hip, knee, and ankle: Blue dots. **Joint Moment Arm:** Perpendicular distance from AOR to GRFV.
RESULTANT EXTERNAL MOMENTS
• **Hip: Extension**—GRFV is visualized posterior to hip AOR. Resisted passively by anterior hip structures. • **Knee: Extension**—GRFV is visualized anterior to knee AOR. Resisted passively by posterior knee structures. • **Ankle: DF**—GRFV is visualized anterior to ankle AOR. Resisted actively primarily by the S muscle.
COM: center of mass; AOR: axis of rotation; S: soleus

Frontal Plane

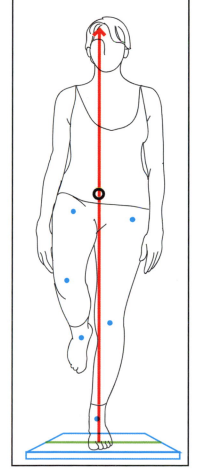

Figure 4-5. Quiet standing (one legged stance) frontal plane with GRFV visualization.

TABLE 4-3. FRONTAL PLANE GROUND REACTION FORCE VECTOR VISUALIZATION
VISUALIZING THE EXTERNAL MOMENT IN THE FRONTAL PLANE DURING SINGLE LIMB STANDING
GRFV depicts the resultant vertical and M/L forces the floor imposes on the body (red line).
COM FOR THE BODY: BLACK CIRCLE
AOR for the hip, knee, and ankle: Blue dots.   **Joint Moment Arm:** Perpendicular distance from AOR to GRFV.
RESULTANT EXTERNAL MOMENTS
<ul><li>**Hip: Adduction**—GRFV is visualized medial to the AOR. Resisted actively by gluteus medius and minimus.</li><li>**Knee: Varus/Adduction**—GRFV is visualized medial to AOR. Resisted passively by lateral knee structures.</li><li>**Ankle: Eversion**—GRFV is visualized lateral to AOR. Resisted actively by tibialis anterior, tibialis posterior, and S muscles.</li></ul>

4.3: CENTER OF PRESSURE

Quiet Stance

Center of Pressure (COP) represents the net moments acting within the BOS, and is visualized as the intersection of the GRFV with the floor. During quiet stance, the A/P and lateral coordinates of the COP and COM coincide because there is little movement.[3] Once dynamic motion occurs, they follow opposite trajectories.[3,4] The COM is located in the pelvis, while the COP is a single point within the BOS. The COP's location in quiet stance is visualized for the total base of support, rather than under each foot as depicted during single limb support in walking. Its average location is slightly left of midline (0.57 cm), anterior to the ankle axis, and posterior to the metatarsophalangeal axis creating an external ankle DF moment.[4,5] The ankle plantar flexor muscles control the external moment caused by the COM's anterior position.[4]

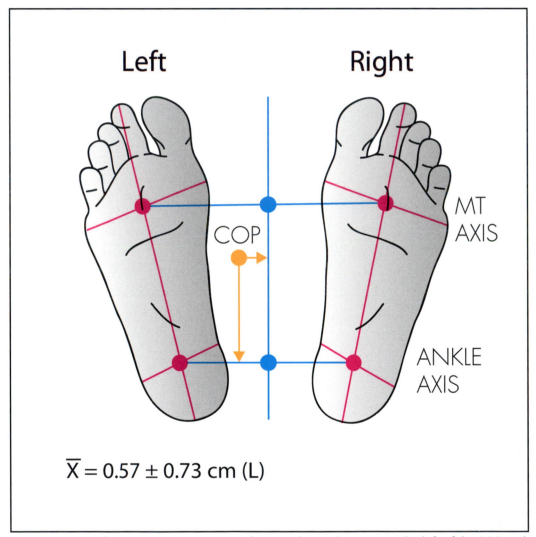

Figure 4-6. COP location during quiet standing. It is located 0.57 cm to the left of the BOS midline. (Adapted from Adams J. *Quanitative assessment of static and dynamic postural stability in normal adults* [thesis]. Los Angeles: Department of Biokinesiology and Physical Therapy, at University of Southern California; 1987.)

During Gait Initiation

Gait initiation is characterized by a series of controlled postural shifts that culminate in a forward step. When initiating a step with the right limb during quiet stance, the COP first moves rapidly in a posterior direction toward the right foot (swing limb).[3,4,6,7] The COM, which is located in the trunk is simultaneously moving anteriorly towards the stance limb.[3,4] As the right limb begins unloading, the COP then moves laterally towards the left (stance limb).[3] Once right toe off occurs, the COP moves anteriorly toward the metatarsal heads, and finally moves under the toes as the left (stance) limb is unloaded.[3,6] The trajectory of the COP varies little between individuals regardless of the speed at which gait is initiated, so it is characterized as a stereotypical pattern.[3,4] According to Jian et al,[3] steady state gait is achieved at the end of the second step at normal speeds, in contrast to the first step as suggested by Breniere and Do.[7]

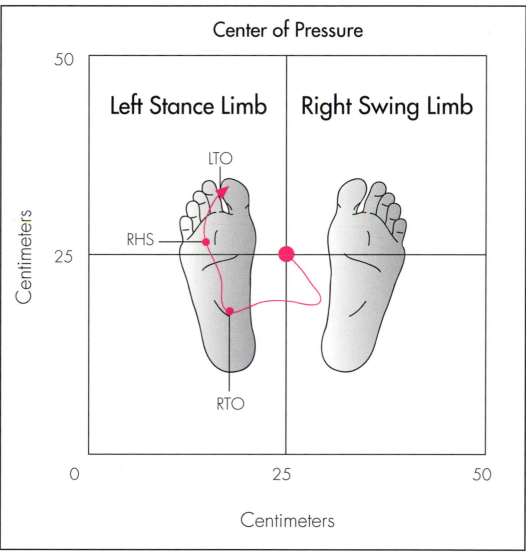

Figure 4-7. COP trajectory during gait initiation with the right limb.

4.4: Ground Reaction Forces During Walking

The 3 components of each limb's GRF, each representing a different orthogonal direction (eg, vertical, anterior/posterior, medio/lateral), are typically measured by a force plate embedded in the walking surface. The force represents the floor's force on the body, which according to Newton's third law is equal in magnitude, but opposite in direction to the body's force on the floor. Since F = M x A, the vertical GRF is greater than body weight due to the acceleration of the body towards the floor during loading.

The force is typically normalized by body weight (Newton [N]/Body Weight [BW]).

Vertical: **Maximum ~ 110% BW in early Mid Stance/late Terminal GRF Stance**
Minimum ~ 70% BW in late Mid Stance/early Terminal Stance

A/P: **Maximum Posterior ~ 20% BW in Loading Response/Mid GRF Stance**
Maximum Anterior ~ 20% BW in Terminal Stance/Pre-Swing

M/L: **Maximum Medial ~ 5% BW in single limb support GRF**

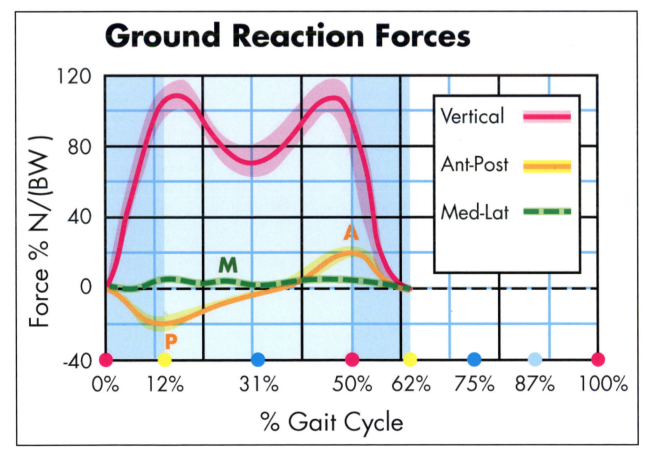

Figure 4-8. Normalized GRF (N/BW).

4.5: SAGITTAL PLANE KINETICS DURING STANCE PHASE

Initial Contact

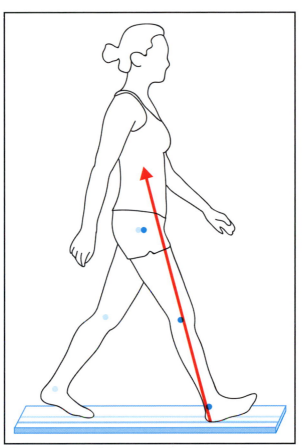

Figure 4-9. Initial Contact with GRFV visualization.

TABLE 4-4. INITIAL CONTACT: EXTERNAL MOMENTS WITH MUSCLE ACTIVATION			
JOINT/SEGMENT	**GRFV VISUALIZATION**	**EXTERNAL MOMENTS**	**MUSCLE ACTIVITY**
Ankle	Posterior	PF	Dorsiflexors
Knee	Anterior	Extension	Vasti
Hip	Anterior	Flexion	Hip extensors

Loading Response

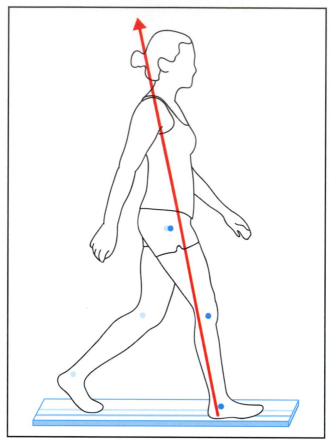

Figure 4-10. Loading Response with GRFV visualization.

TABLE 4-5. LOADING RESPONSE: EXTERNAL MOMENTS WITH MUSCLE ACTIVATION			
JOINT/SEGMENT	GRFV VISUALIZATION	EXTERNAL MOMENTS	MUSCLE ACTIVITY
Ankle	Posterior	PF	Dorsiflexors
Knee	Posterior	Flexion	Vasti
Hip	Anterior	Flexion	Hip extensors

Mid Stance

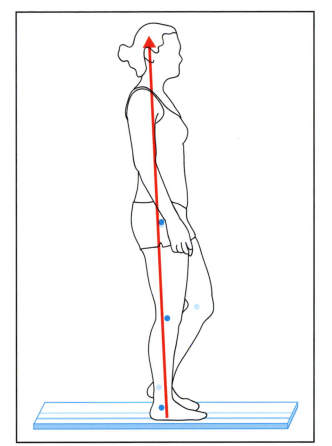

Figure 4-11. Mid Stance with GRFV visualization.

TABLE 4-6. MID STANCE: EXTERNAL MOMENTS WITH MUSCLE ACTIVATION			
JOINT/SEGMENT	**GRFV VISUALIZATION**	**EXTERNAL MOMENTS**	**MUSCLE ACTIVITY**
Ankle	Anterior	DF	Plantar flexors
Knee	Posterior to Anterior	Flexion to extension	Vasti during flexion moment, no activity during extension moment
Hip	Anterior to Posterior	Flexion to extension	No activity

Terminal Stance

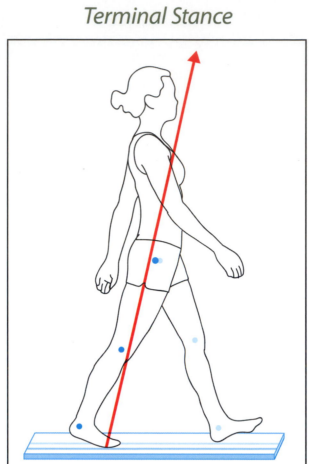

Figure 4-12. Terminal Stance with GRFV visualization.

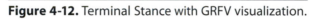

TABLE 4-7. TERMINAL STANCE: EXTERNAL MOMENTS WITH MUSCLE ACTIVATION			
JOINT/SEGMENT	**GRFV VISUALIZATION**	**EXTERNAL MOMENTS**	**MUSCLE ACTIVITY**
Ankle	Anterior	DF	Plantar flexors
Knee	Anterior, moves posterior just before CL IC	Extension, flexion just before CL IC	None
Hip	Posterior	Extension	None
CL IC: contralateral Initial Contact			

Pre-Swing

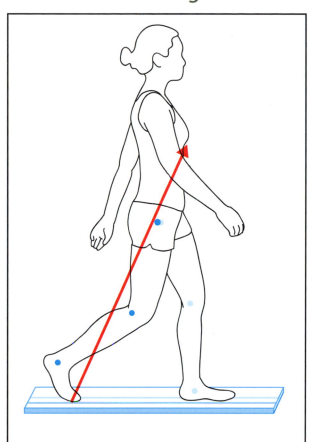

Figure 4-13. Pre-Swing with GRFV visualization.

TABLE 4-8. PRE-SWING: EXTERNAL MOMENTS WITH MUSCLE ACTIVATION			
JOINT/SEGMENT	**GRFV VISUALIZATION**	**EXTERNAL MOMENTS**	**MUSCLE ACTIVITY**
Ankle	Anterior	DF	Elastic recoil of plantar flexors
Knee	Posterior	Flexion	Rectus femoris
Hip	Posterior	Decreasing extension	Adductor longus, and rectus femoris

4.6: Sagittal Plane Moments by Joint

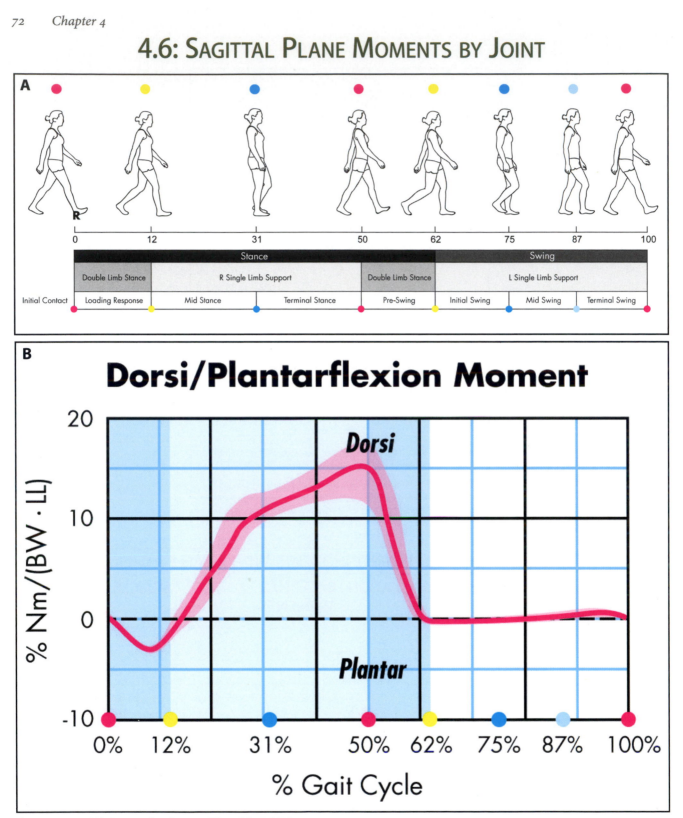

Figure 4-14. (A) Gait cycle phases. (B) Ankle DF/PF moments.

TABLE 4-9	
PHASES	**EXTERNAL SAGITTAL ANKLE MOMENTS[8]**
Initial Contact and Loading Response:	**Minimal PF Moment** • Eccentric dorsiflexor activity peaks to control PF and initiate forward movement of the tibia, contributing to knee flexion (AT, extensor digitorum longus, and extensor hallucis longus)
Mid Stance:	**DF Moment** • Eccentric S, G, FDL, and FHL activity • Eccentric PT and fibularis (FL and FB) activity
Terminal Stance:	**Peak DF Moment** • Highest activity of S, G, FDL and FHL • Concentric PT and eccentric fibularis activity
Pre-Swing:	**Decreasing DF Moment** • Early plantar flexor activity quickly ceases • Elastic recoil of the plantar flexors continues to diminish DF moment as ankle plantar flexes • Onset of dorsiflexor activity prepares for swing DF clearance
Initial Swing, Mid Swing, and Terminal Swing:	**Minimal PF Moment** • Dorsiflexor activity brings the ankle to neutral by Mid Swing for foot clearance
AT: anterior tibialis; FDL: flexor digitorum longus; FHL: flexor hallucis longus; PT: posterior tibialis; FL: fibularis longus; FB: fibularis brevis	

4.7: ANKLE DORSIFLEXOR EMG WITH MOMENTS

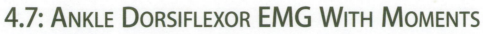

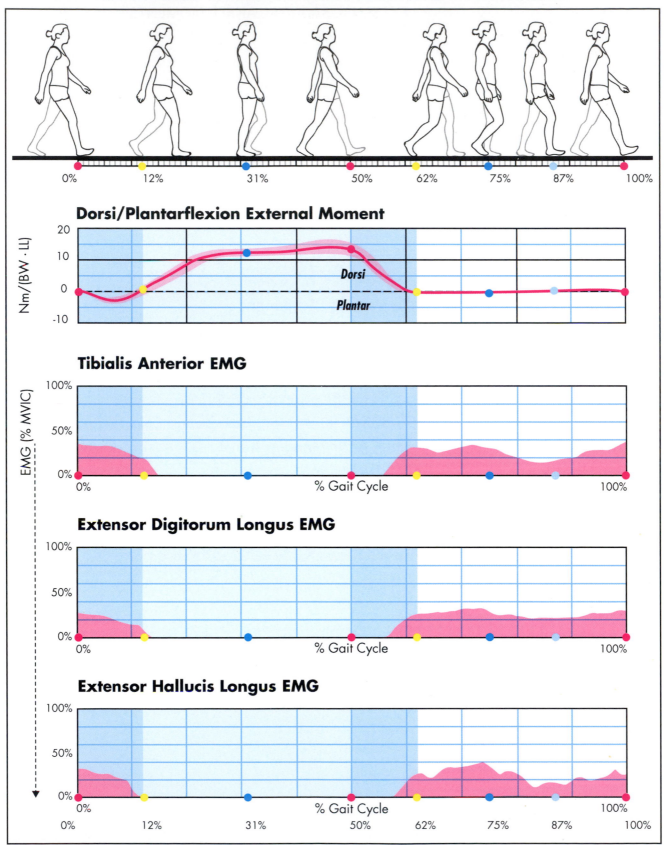

Figure 4-15. Ankle dorsiflexor EMG with external moments.

4.8: ANKLE PLANTAR FLEXOR EMG WITH MOMENTS

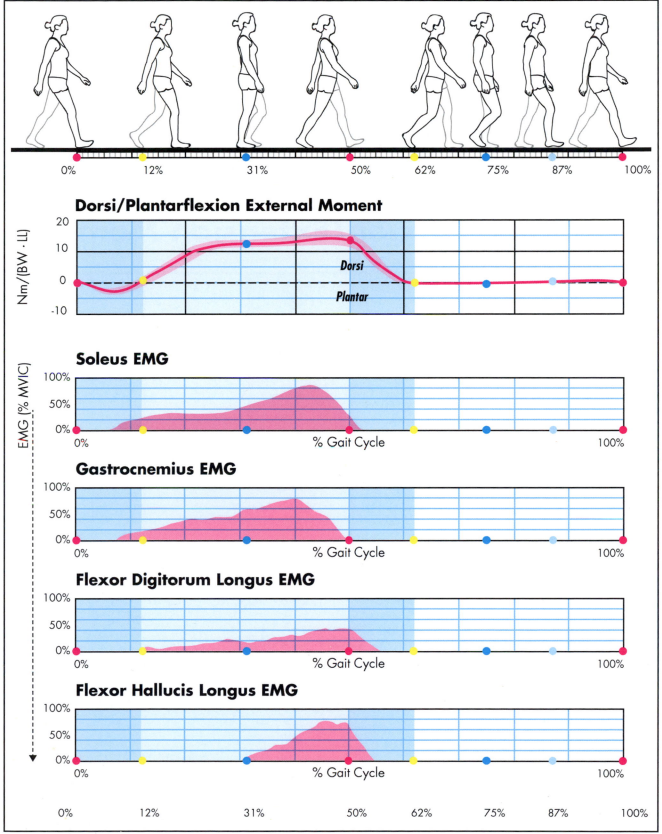

Figure 4-16. Ankle plantar flexor EMG with external moments.

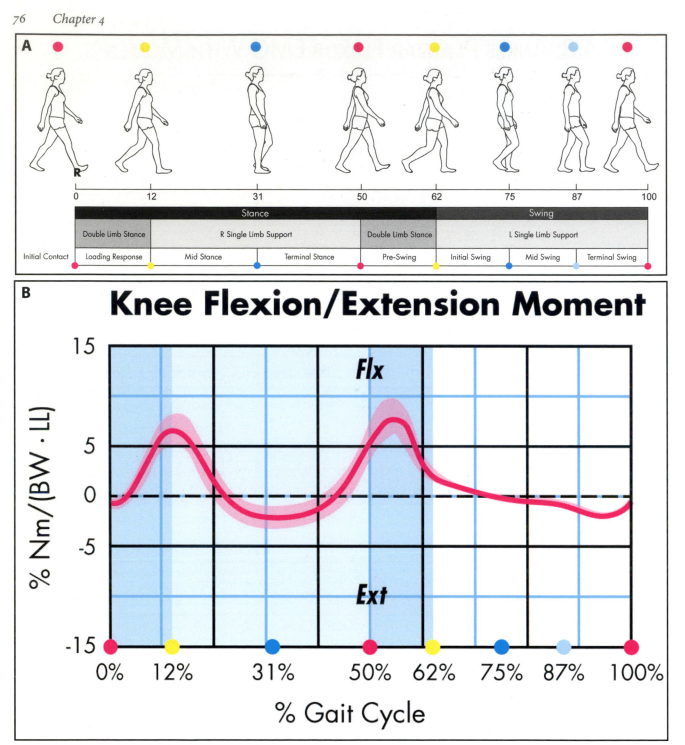

Figure 4-17. (A) Gait cycle phases. (B) Knee flexion/extension moments.

TABLE 4-10	
PHASES	**EXTERNAL SAGITTAL KNEE MOMENTS[8]**
Initial Contact:	**Extension Moment** • Vasti remain active (VMO, VML, VI, VL) in preparation for loading
Loading Response:	**Flexion Moment** • Vasti eccentric activity (VMO, VML, VI, VL)
Mid Stance:	**Decreasing flexion moment and then becomes an extension moment** • The vasti extend knee, but cease activity when GRFV moves anterior to the knee.
Terminal Stance:	**Decreasing extension moment and then an increasing flexion moment that initiates Pre-Swing knee flexion**
Pre-Swing and Initial Swing:	**Flexion Moment** • Rectus femoris eccentric activity to decelerate knee flexion
Terminal Swing:	**Extension Moment** • Vasti activity (VMO, VML, VI, VL) in preparation for Initial Contact and Loading Response, and to counteract the hamstring activity decelerating the limb
VMO: vastus medialis oblique; VML: vastus medialis longus; VI: vastus intermedius; VL: vastus lateralis	

4.9: KNEE EXTENSOR EMG WITH MOMENTS

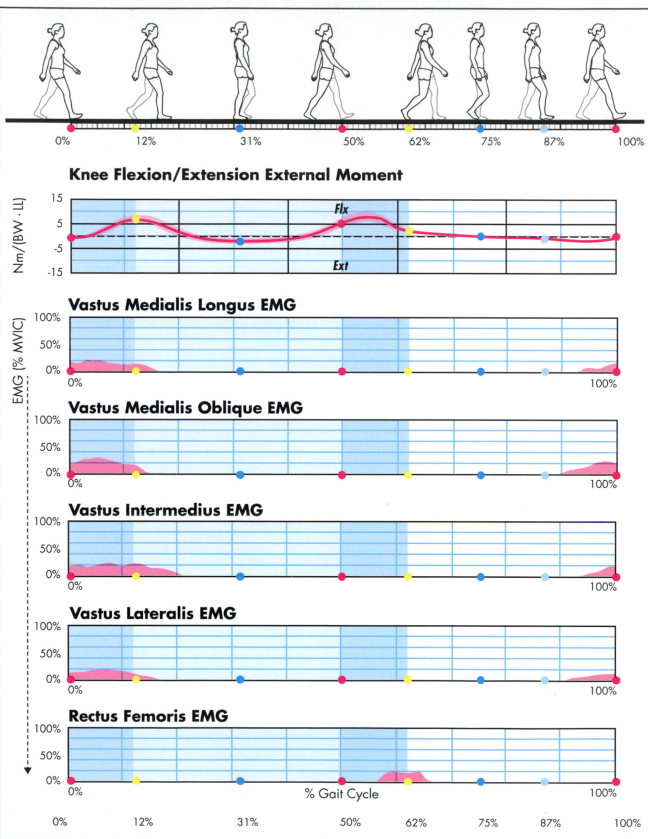

Figure 4-18. Knee extensor EMG with external moments.

4.10: KNEE FLEXOR EMG WITH MOMENTS

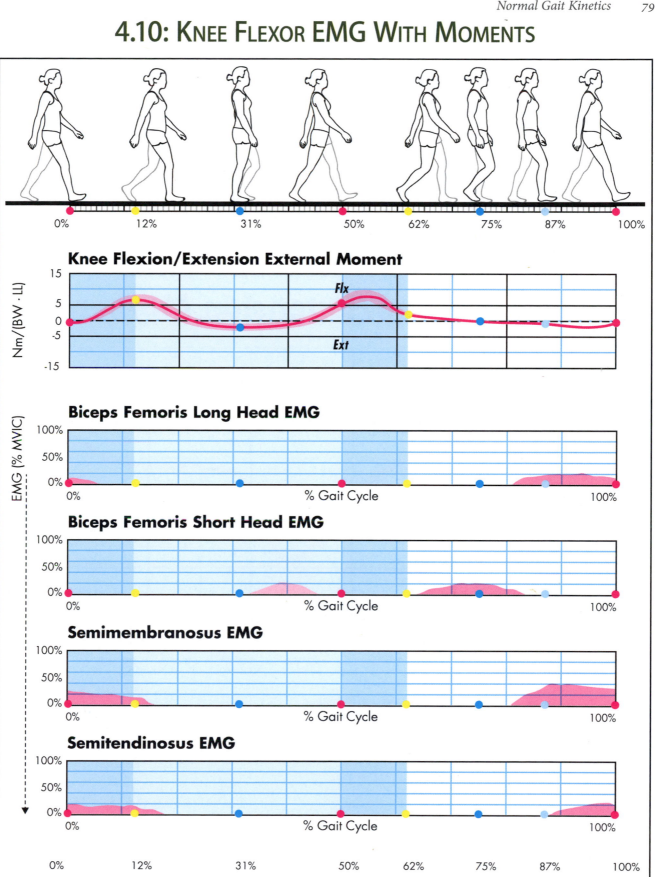

Figure 4-19. Knee flexor EMG with external moments.

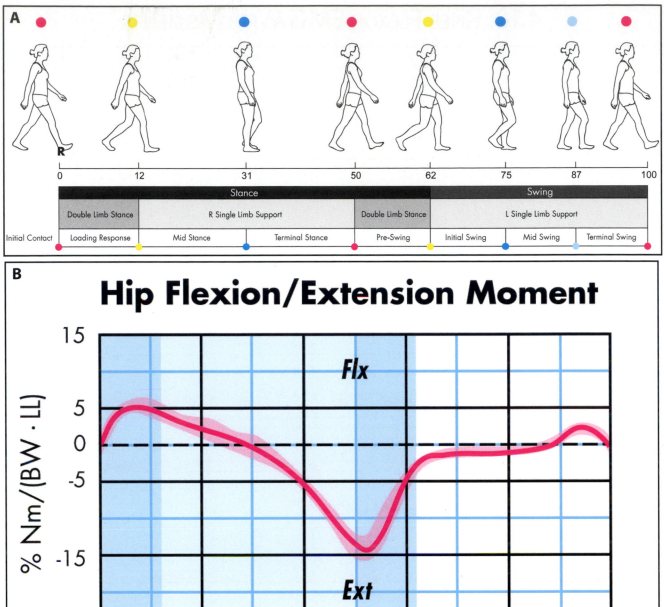

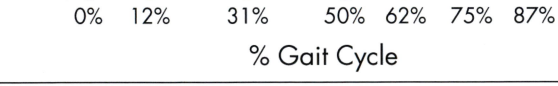

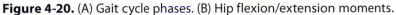

Figure 4-20. (A) Gait cycle phases. (B) Hip flexion/extension moments.

TABLE 4-11	
PHASES	**EXTERNAL SAGITTAL HIP MOMENTS[8]**
Initial Contact and Loading Response:	**Flexion Moment** • Hip extensor activity (upper and lower g-max, adductor magnus, SM, ST, LHBF)
Mid Stance:	**Early Flexion Moment** **Extension Moment** • Passively resisted by the anterior hip structures as the hip is extending by momentum
Terminal Stance:	**Extension Moment** • Passively resisted by the anterior hip structures
Pre-Swing, Initial Swing, and Mid Swing:	**Decreasing Extension Moment** • Adductor longus initiates hip flexion in Pre-Swing, the rectus femoris activates later in Pre-Swing to flex the hip while limiting knee flexion. The Iliacus and sartorius are active during Initial and Mid Swing. The LHBF and SM activity in late Mid Swing decelerate the limb in preparation for Initial Contact.
Terminal Swing:	**Flexion Moment** • Hip extensor activity to decelerate limb to prepare for Initial Contact (upper and lower g-max, adductor magnus, SM, ST, LHBF)
g-max: gluteus maximus; SM: semimembranosus; ST: semitendinosus; LHBF: long head biceps femoris	

4.11: HIP EXTENSOR EMG WITH MOMENTS

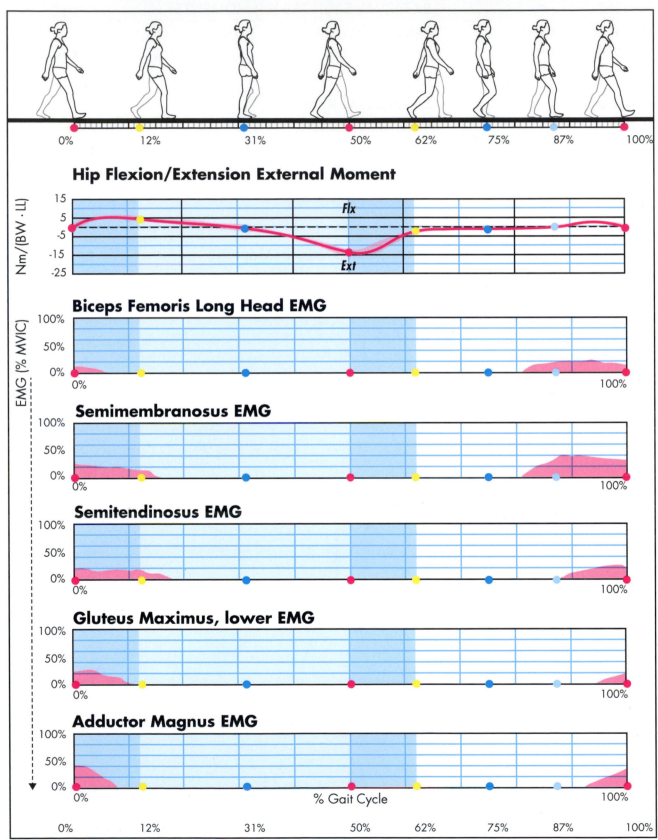

Figure 4-21. Hip extensor EMG with external moments.

4.12: HIP FLEXOR EMG WITH MOMENTS

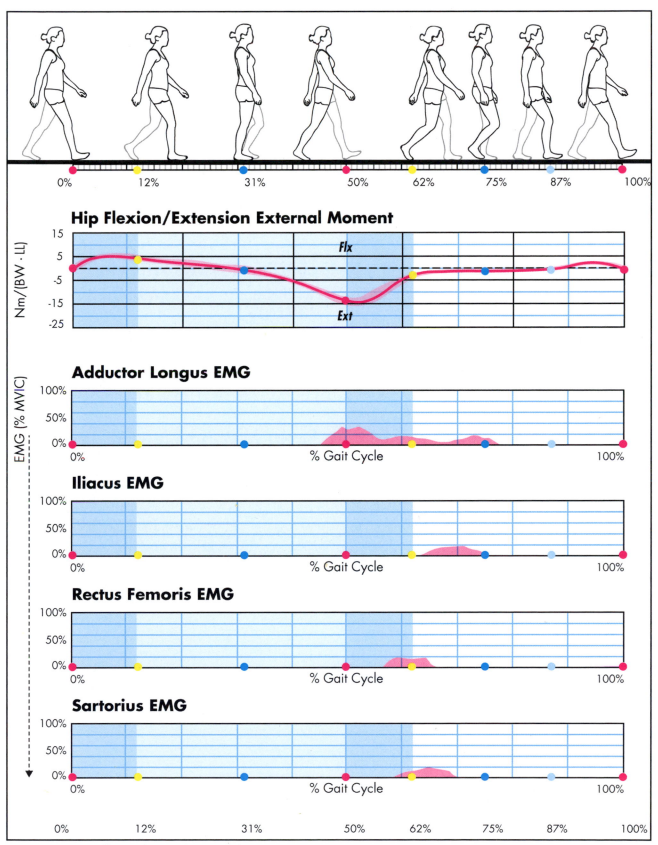

Figure 4-22. Hip flexor EMG with external moments.

4.13: Frontal Plane Kinetics

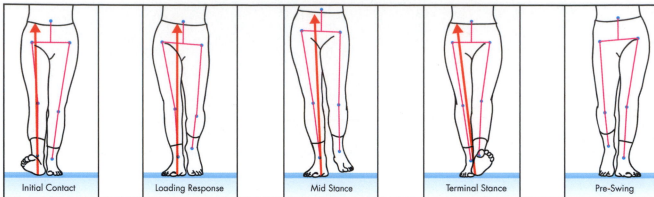

| Initial Contact | Loading Response | Mid Stance | Terminal Stance | Pre-Swing |

Figure 4-23. Frontal plane figures with GRFV visualization.

Table 4-12. Initial Contact and Loading Moments With EMG

JOINT/SEGMENT	GRFV VISUALIZATION	EXTERNAL MOMENTS	MUSCLE ACTIVITY
Subtalar	Lateral	Eversion	Invertors (AT and PT)
Knee	Medial	Varus	None
Hip	Medial	Adduction	Abductors

Table 4-13. Mid and Terminal Stance Moments With EMG

JOINT/SEGMENT	GRFV VISUALIZATION	EXTERNAL MOMENTS	MUSCLE ACTIVITY
Subtalar	Lateral to medial	Eversion to inversion	Evertors and PF (FL, FB, PT, FHL, FDL, S, G)
Knee	Medial	Varus	None
Hip	Medial	Adduction	Abductors

4.14: CALCANEAL KINEMATICS AND INVERTOR/EVERTOR MUSCLE ACTIVITY

Note: In observational analysis the evaluator is observing the calcaneal position in reference to the tibia, which is not true subtalar motion (talus and calcaneus). Therefore, during observational analysis the calcaneal/tibial angle is evaluated, which in part describes the triplanar subtalar motion that primarily occurs in the frontal plane. We have included the kinematics coupled with muscle activity (EMG).

Invertor/Evertor EMG

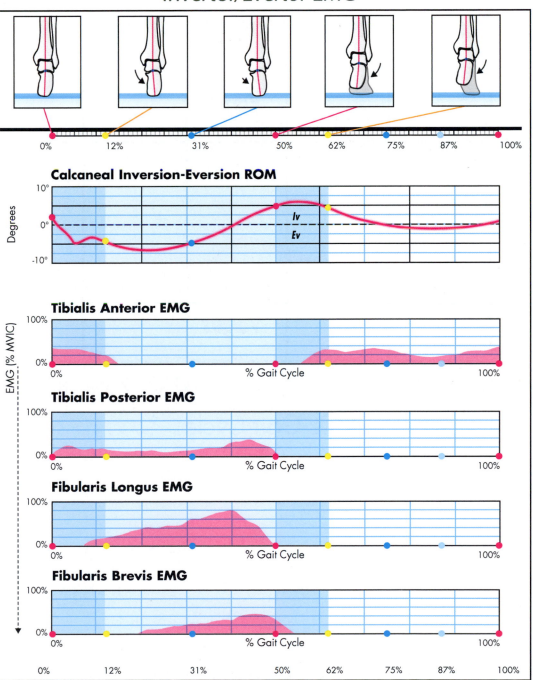

Figure 4-24. Invertor/evertor EMG with calcaneal kinematics.

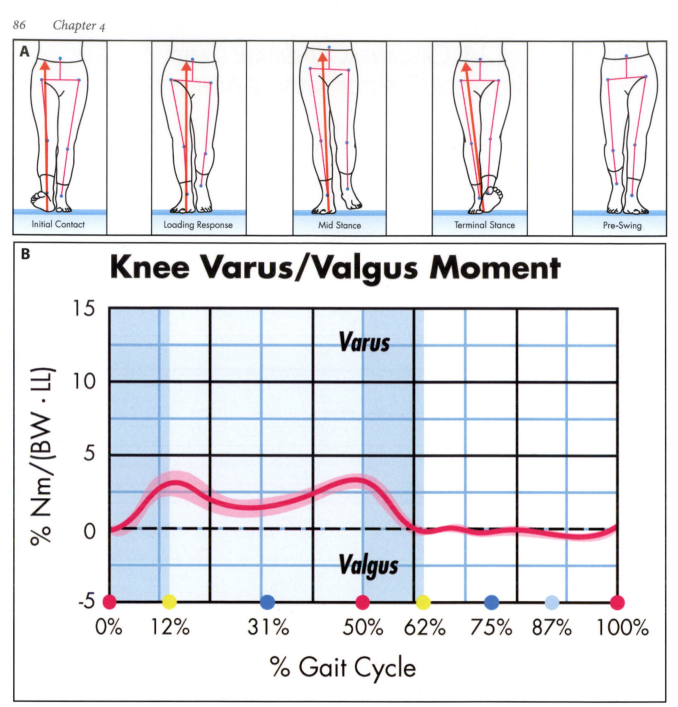

Figure 4-25. (A) Frontal view with vector. (B) Frontal plane knee varus/valgus moments.

TABLE 4-14	
PHASES	EXTERNAL KNEE FRONTAL MOMENTS
Initial Contact:	Neutral Moment
Loading Response:	Neutral to Increasing Varus/Adduction Moment • Resisted passively by lateral knee structures
Mid Stance:	Varus/Adduction Moment • Resisted passively by lateral knee structures
Terminal Stance:	Varus/Adduction Moment • Resisted passively by lateral knee structures
Pre-Swing:	Varus/Adduction Moment Decreases to Neutral
Initial Swing, Mid Swing, and Terminal Swing:	Neutral Moment • Slight valgus/abduction moment decreases to neutral by Initial Contact

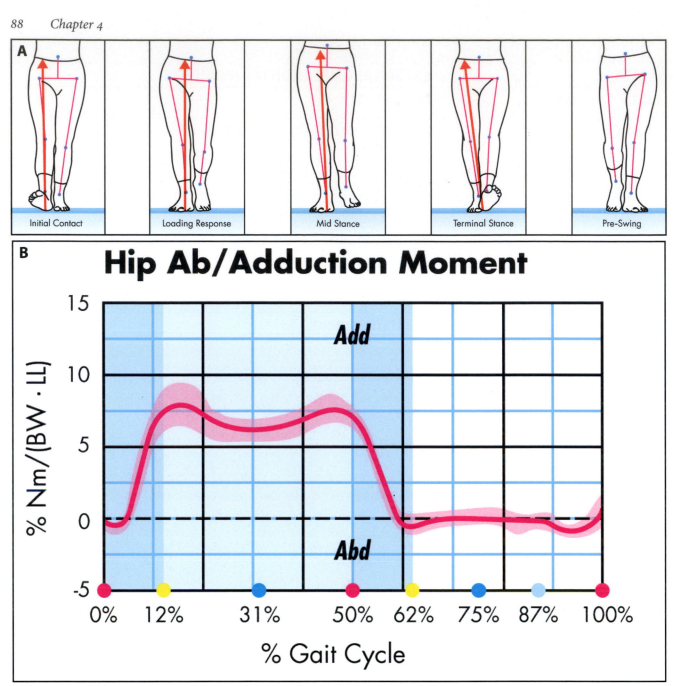

Figure 4-26. (A) Frontal view with vector. (B) Frontal plane hip abduction/adduction moments.

TABLE 4-15	
PHASES	**EXTERNAL HIP FRONTAL MOMENTS**
Initial Contact:	Neutral Moment • Hip abductor activity in preparation for Loading Response (upper and lower g-max, g-med, TFL)
Loading Response:	Increasing Adduction Moment • Eccentric hip abductor activity to minimize contralateral pelvic drop (upper and lower g-max, g-med, and TFL)
Mid Stance:	Peak Adduction Moment • Eccentric hip abductor activity to minimize contralateral pelvic drop (upper g-max, g-med, and TFL)
Terminal Stance:	Second Peak Adduction Moment • TFL activity to maintain a level pelvis
Pre-Swing:	Adduction Moment Decreases • Adduction moment rapidly decreasing to neutral as the limb is unloaded
Initial Swing, Mid Swing, and Terminal Swing:	Neutral Moment
g-med: gluteus medius; TFL: tensor fascia lata	

Hip Abductor EMG

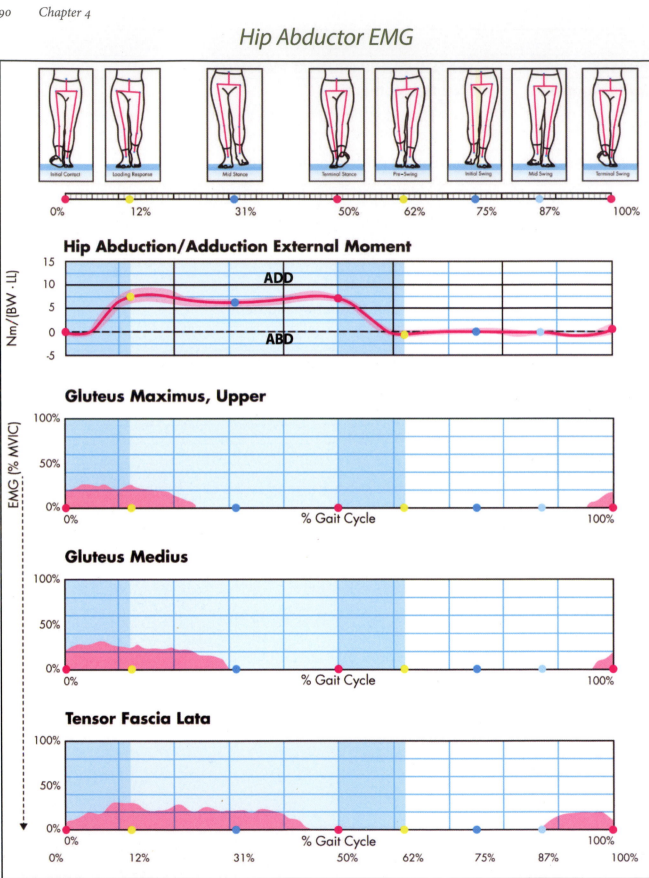

Figure 4-27. Hip abductor EMG with external moments.

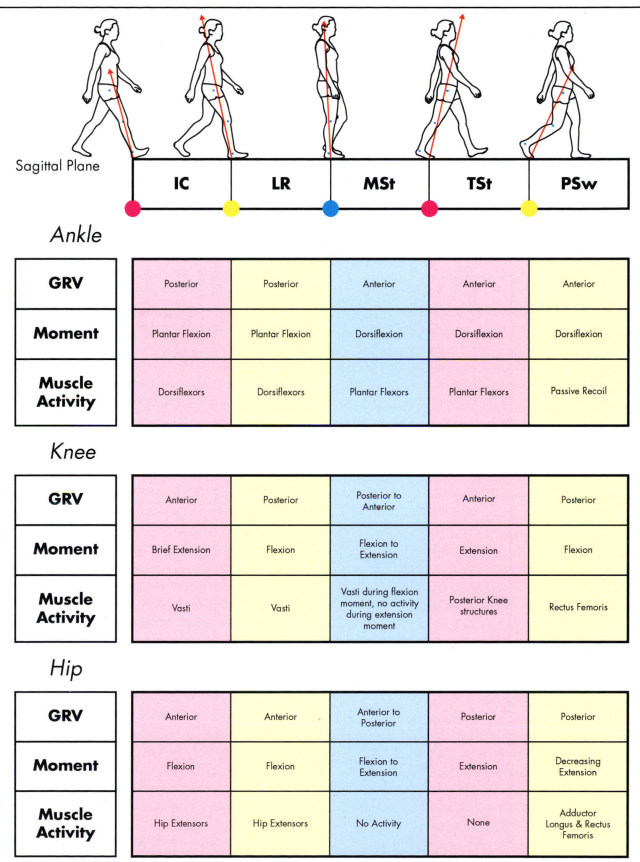

Sagittal Plane	IC	LR	MSt	TSt	PSw

Ankle

	IC	LR	MSt	TSt	PSw
GRV	Posterior	Posterior	Anterior	Anterior	Anterior
Moment	Plantar Flexion	Plantar Flexion	Dorsiflexion	Dorsiflexion	Dorsiflexion
Muscle Activity	Dorsiflexors	Dorsiflexors	Plantar Flexors	Plantar Flexors	Passive Recoil

Knee

	IC	LR	MSt	TSt	PSw
GRV	Anterior	Posterior	Posterior to Anterior	Anterior	Posterior
Moment	Brief Extension	Flexion	Flexion to Extension	Extension	Flexion
Muscle Activity	Vasti	Vasti	Vasti during flexion moment, no activity during extension moment	Posterior Knee structures	Rectus Femoris

Hip

	IC	LR	MSt	TSt	PSw
GRV	Anterior	Anterior	Anterior to Posterior	Posterior	Posterior
Moment	Flexion	Flexion	Flexion to Extension	Extension	Decreasing Extension
Muscle Activity	Hip Extensors	Hip Extensors	No Activity	None	Adductor Longus & Rectus Femoris

Figure 4-28. Summary table for stance phase sagittal moments and muscle activity.

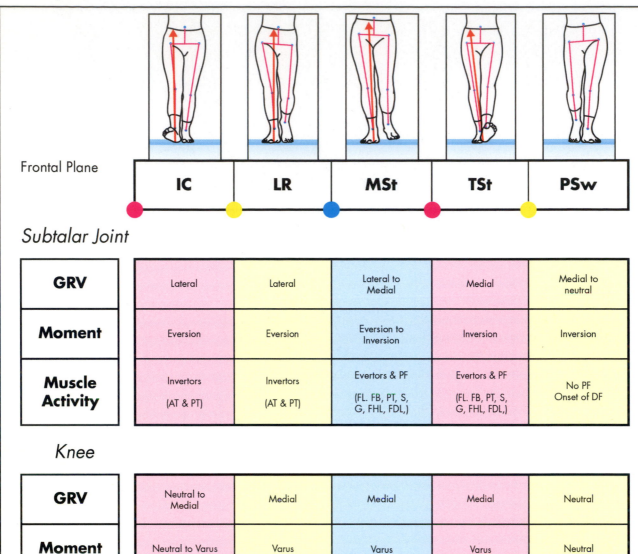

Frontal Plane

	IC	LR	MSt	TSt	PSw

Subtalar Joint

	IC	LR	MSt	TSt	PSw
GRV	Lateral	Lateral	Lateral to Medial	Medial	Medial to neutral
Moment	Eversion	Eversion	Eversion to Inversion	Inversion	Inversion
Muscle Activity	Invertors (AT & PT)	Invertors (AT & PT)	Evertors & PF (FL. FB, PT, S, G, FHL, FDL,)	Evertors & PF (FL. FB, PT, S, G, FHL, FDL,)	No PF Onset of DF

Knee

	IC	LR	MSt	TSt	PSw
GRV	Neutral to Medial	Medial	Medial	Medial	Neutral
Moment	Neutral to Varus	Varus	Varus	Varus	Neutral
Muscle Activity	None	None	None	None	None

Hip

	IC	LR	MSt	TSt	PSw
GRV	Neutral to Medial	Medial	Medial	Medial	Medial to Neutral
Moment	Adduction	Adduction	Adduction	Adduction	Neutral
Muscle Activity	Abductors (U G-max, G-med, G-min, TFL)	Abductors (U G-max, G-med, G-min, TFL)	Abductors (U G-max, G-med, G-min, TFL)	Abductor (TFL)	None

Figure 4-29. Summary table for stance phase frontal moments and muscle activity.

> *i* All figures in this chapter except Figures 4-1, 4-2, 4-3, 4-4, 4-5, 4-7, 4-8, 4-14, 4-17, 4-20, and 4-25 are adapted from Perry J, Burnfield JM. *Gait Analysis: Normal & Pathological Gait*. 2nd ed. Thorofare, NJ: SLACK Incorporated; 2010; Kadaba MP, Ramakrishnan HK, Wootten ME, Gainey J, Gorton G, Cochran GV. Repeatability of kinematic, kinetic, and electromyographic data in normal adult gait. *J Orthop Res*. 1989;7[6]:849-860.

4.15: REFERENCES

1. Whittington B, Silder A, Heiderscheit B, Thelen DG. The contribution of passive-elastic mechanisms to lower extremity joint kinetics during human walking. *Gait Posture*. 2008;27(4):628-634.
2. Fukunaga T, Kubo K, Kawakami Y, Fukashiro S, Kanehisa H, Maganaris CN. In vivo behaviour of human muscle tendon during walking. *Proc Biol Sci*. 2001;268(1464):229-233.
3. Jian Y, Winter D, Ishac M, Gilchrist L. Trajectory of the body COG and COP during initiation and termination of gait. *Gait Posture*. 1993;1(1):9-22.
4. Elble RJ, Moody C, Leffler K, Sinha R. The initiation of normal walking. *Mov Disord*. 1994;9(2):139-146.
5. Adams J. *Quanitative assessment of static and dynamic postural stability in normal adults* [thesis]. Los Angeles: Department of Biokinesiology and Physical Therapy, at University of Southern California; 1987.
6. Breniere Y, Do MC. Control of gait initiation. *J Mot Behav*. 1991;23(4):235-240.
7. Breniere Y, Do MC. When and how does steady state gait movement induced from upright posture begin? *J Biomech*. 1986;19(12):1035-1040.
8. Kadaba MP, Ramakrishnan HK, Wootten ME, Gainey J, Gorton G, Cochran GV. Repeatability of kinematic, kinetic, and electromyographic data in normal adult gait. *J Orthop Res*. 1989;7(6):849-860.

Please see videos on the accompanying website at

www.healio.com/books/oga

Chapter 5

Functional Gait Measures

Olfat Mohamed, PhD, PT

A myriad of gait-specific, activity-based, functional measures have been developed to evaluate and quantify complex tasks required to participate in community life. These functional measures are useful in documenting the participant's current status, change over time, and response to interventions. Complex, gait-specific tasks include: walking at a safe speed to cross street intersections; accelerating and decelerating walking pace as needed; negotiating varying terrains; navigating around obstacles; orienting the head in multiple directions; as well as the ability to stop, turn, and change directions. Multitasking items reflects higher level accomplishments.

While *Observational Gait Analysis* identifies phase-specific gait deviations from normal, functional measures provide information about how these deviations affect the participants' ability to meet mobility demands in their environment. Most functional measures require no specialized equipment, which makes them practical to perform in most settings. Most of these measures can be used in multiple diagnostic groups including those with musculoskeletal, neurological, and cardiopulmonary disorders. In this chapter, the most common gait-specific functional measures are described and evaluated.

Scores for functional measures are usually compared to previously established performance levels or *normative* data, which characterizes the full spectrum of a specific population. Normative values are not always available in the literature because of the complex research designs required to establish these data. The term *reference values* signifies the normative values for a specific diagnostic population.

Psychometric properties are quantifiable qualities related to the statistical strength or weakness of a clinical measure. The usefulness of a functional measure in clinical decision making depends on its psychometric properties, which include reliability, validity, and responsiveness.

5.1: RELIABILITY

Reliability is the extent to which a consistent score is obtained on different administrations of the instrument, when all relevant conditions remain essentially constant. Types of reliability include whether the test was repeated at a different time (test-retest), by the same rater (intrarater), or multiple raters (interrater).

Assessing reliability using correlation coefficients (eg, Pearson or Spearman coefficients) is not desirable as it provides the degree of association between 2 scores, but does not address agreement between them. In addition, correlation coefficients are limited to comparing 2 ratings only and not applicable to multiple comparisons. The intraclass correlation coefficients (ICC), on the other hand, reflect both association and agreement among multiple ratings. For the purpose of this chapter, we have adopted the guidelines suggested by the reviewers of the Rehabilitation Measures Database[1] for all psychometric measures.

The strength of the ICC is considered as follows:

ICC > 0.75	**Excellent**
ICC = 0.40 to 0.74	**Adequate**
ICC < 0.40	**Poor**

Adams JM, Cerny K.
Observational Gait Analysis: A Visual Guide (pp 95-141).
© 2018 SLACK Incorporated.

5.2: Validity

Validity assures that a test is measuring what it is intended to measure. It is essential when deciding how the test/measure can be used. Several types of validity exist for most clinical measures, however, for the purpose of this chapter only concurrent validity is addressed because of its objectivity and direct application to clinical practice.

Concurrent validity indicates the strength of association and direction of the relationship between the scores of the test of interest and another test that is considered the "gold standard," or a test with established validity. The 2 tests are usually conducted at relatively the same time. Relationships between the scores are commonly expressed using the Pearson product-moment correlation coefficient (r) for ratio and interval scales, while the Kappa and the Spearman rank correlation coefficient (r_s), also called Spearman's rho, are used for nominal and ordinal data. Unless rated by the author(s), the strength of the relationship is considered as follows:

Correlation coefficient > 0.6	**Excellent**
Correlation coefficient = 0.30 to 0.59	**Adequate**
Correlation coefficient < 0.30	**Poor**

5.3: Minimal Detectable Change

Responsiveness to change, which is the ability of the functional measure to accurately detect change, when in fact change has occurred, is commonly evaluated through the calculation of the minimal detectable change (MDC). The MDC is the smallest change in the participant's score that represents a true change beyond measurement error.

Although the MDC defines the magnitude of what is considered a real change in measurement score, it is important to determine if this change is actually meaningful in the participant's response. For example, it is unlikely that a 0.5-second improvement in the Timed Up and Go (TUG) test indicates a meaningful difference in the participants' function.

5.4: Minimal Clinically Important Difference

The most common indicator of meaningful change is called the minimal clinically important difference (MCID). The MCID, represents the minimum change in the score that reflects meaningful change perceived by the participant or the clinician as noticeable improvement in performance.

Responsiveness may also be reflected through the calculation of the effect size (ES), the standardized response mean (SRM), or both. The value of using the ES or SRM is the ability to compare responsiveness of different functional measures with varying measurement scales. As a general rule, large effect size indicates a larger treatment effect. Thus, ES in the 0.90s and 0.80s is considered large, while ES in the 0.20s is considered minimal.

5.5: Cut-Off Scores

Cut-off scores on functional measures help categorize participants into groups. For example, a cut-off score of 10/12 on the 4-Item Dynamic Gait Index indicates that the participant is at risk for falls.

For more data on any of these functional measures the reader is encouraged to consult the Rehabilitation Measures website.[1]

5.6: The Timed Up and Go Test

Link to the Instrument:

http://www.rehabmeasures.org/PDF%20Library/Timed%20Up%20and%20Go%20Test%20Instructions.pdf

Purpose

The original purpose of the TUG test was to test general mobility and fall risk in frail, elderly people.[2] It has been used with other populations, including people with arthritis, Parkinson's disease, vestibular problems, and people who have suffered a stroke. The American Geriatric Society and the British Geriatric Society guidelines recommend the TUG as a routine screening test for falls.[3]

Description

The test requires the subject to rise from sitting in a standard arm chair, walk 3 m to a target mark or a cone, turn around the mark/cone (180 degrees), walk back to the chair, and sit down; moving as quickly and safely as possible. The score is the time between the command to start, till the buttocks touch the seat of the chair. The participant should have one practice trial that is not included in the score.[2]

Scoring

Time in seconds

Area of Assessment

Balance (vestibular and nonvestibular), functional mobility, and gait

ICF Domain

Activity

Time to Administer

Five minutes or less

Equipment

- Standard armchair (approximately 46 cm in height)
- A cone or other mark of distance
- A stop watch

Reference Values

Several studies reported reference ranges for the TUG in community-dwelling older adults, with consistently longer average times with increasing age and for women compared to men.[4-7] Bohannon, using a meta-analysis, consolidated data from 21 studies that reported TUG reference values in people older than 60 years of age (Table 5.6.1).[5]

TABLE 5.6.1. TIMED UP AND GO REFERENCE VALUES FOR COMMUNITY-DWELLING, OLDER ADULTS[5]		
AGE (YEARS)	MEAN (SECONDS)	95% CI
60 to 69	8.1	7.1 to 9.0
70 to 79	9.2	8.2 to 10.2
80 to 89	11.3	10.0 to 12.7
CI: confidence interval		

Minimal Detectable Change

TABLE 5.6.2. TIMED UP AND GO MINIMAL DETECTABLE CHANGE VALUES		
DIAGNOSTIC GROUP	MINIMAL DETECTABLE CHANGES (SECONDS)	REFERENCES
Alzheimer's disease	4.09	Ries et al[8]
Chronic stroke	2.9	Flansbjer et al[9]
Parkinson's disease	11.3	Dal Bello-Haas et al[10]

Minimal Clinically Important Difference

Write et al[11] measured the TUG scores at baseline, and then after 9 weeks of physical therapy in a group of patients with hip osteoarthritis. Using 3 different statistical calculation methods they reported that a reduction in the TUG time greater than or equal to 0.8, 1.4, and 1.2 seconds are the MCID.[11]

Cut-Off Scores

Cut-off scores are commonly used to identify individuals at risk for falls. The cut-off score is different in different populations and across different diagnostic groups (Table 5.6.3). For example, using a cut-off score of 20 seconds, the TUG was 87% sensitive and specific in distinguishing older community-dwelling fallers from nonfallers.[12] Clinicians, however, should not rely solely on the TUG to identify fall risk because of the variability reported between studies and populations in cut-off scores as reported in systematic reviews and meta-analyses.[13-16] Furthermore, the TUG is not suitable to identify fallers in high-functioning, older adult populations because it is not challenging enough (ceiling effect).[16] In addition to timing the TUG, clinicians should observe how the individual performs the TUG to gain important clinical insight into the quality of the sit-to-stand, stepping, arm swing, steadiness, ability to turn, etc.

TABLE 5.6.3. CUT-OFF SCORES INDICATING RISK OF FALLS		
POPULATION/ DIAGNOSTIC GROUP	CUT-OFF SCORE (SECONDS)	REFERENCES
Community-dwelling adults	> 13.5	Shumway-Cook et al[12]
Older stoke patients	> 14	Andersson et al[17]
Older adults already attending a falls clinic	> 15	Whitney et al[18]
Frail elderly	> 32.6	Thomas et al[19]
Lower extremity amputees	> 19	Dite et al[20]
Parkinson's disease	> 11.5	Nocera et al[21]
	> 7.95	Dibble et al[22]
Hip osteoarthritis	> 10	Arnold et al[23]
Vestibular disorders	> 11.1	Whitney et al[24]

Psychometric Properties

Test-Retest Reliability

In community-dwelling, older adults, test-retest reliability was excellent with an ICC of 0.97.[7] Test retest reliability is also documented for different diagnostic groups including osteoarthritis (ICC = 0.75),[25] stroke (ICC = 0.96),[9] traumatic brain injury (ICC = 0.86),[26] and Parkinson's disease (ICC = 0.85).[27]

Interrater and Intrarater Reliability

In community-dwelling, older adults with a variety of medical conditions interrater reliability was excellent (ICC = 0.99). Interrater reliability was also excellent in several diagnostic groups including osteoarthritis with ICC = 0.87 (95% CI = 0.74 to 0.94),[11] spinal cord injury (r = 0.973),[28] and Parkinson's disease (ICC = 0.99).[29]

The TUG has demonstrated excellent intrarater reliability as well with ICCs of 0.92 to 0.99.[7,27] Nordin et al[30] tested the intrarater reliability of the TUG in a group of older adults living in a residential care facility in Sweden, and demonstrated excellent intrarater reliability (ICC = 0.92; 95% CI = 0.86 to 0.95). In 20 patients with Parkinson's disease, Bonnie et al[29] reported an ICC of 0.98.

Validity

TABLE 5.6.4. CONCURRENT VALIDITY OF THE TIMED UP AND GO TEST		
POPULATION/ DIAGNOSTIC GROUP	**MEASURES THAT CORRELATE WITH THE TUG**	**REFERENCES**
Older adults with a variety of diagnoses	BBS, $r=-0.81$ Gait speed, $r=-0.61$ Barthel Index of ADL, $r=-0.78$	Podsiadlo et al[2]
	Functional Gait Assessment, $r=-0.84$	Wrisley and Kumar[31]
Parkinson's disease	Berg Balance Scale, $r=-0.78$ Fast gait speed, $r=-0.69$, and comfortable gait speed, $r=-0.67$, in patients with Parkinson's disease.	Brusse et al[32]
	Berg Balance Scale, $r=-0.47$	Bennie et al[29]
Chronic stroke	6MWT, $r=0.92$ Comfortable gait speed, $r=-0.86$ Fast gait speed, $r=-0.91$ Speed of ascending stairs, $r=0.86$ Speed of descending stairs, $r=0.90$	Flansbjer et al[9]
Vestibular disorders	FTSST at baseline measurement, $r=0.53$	Meretta et al[33]
Osteoarthritis	Kellengren-Lawrence radiological stages, $r=0.628$ KOOS, all dimensions, $r=-0.52$ to -0.69	Sabirli et al[34]
Spinal cord injury	SCI-FAI mobility, $r=-0.724$ 10MWT, $r=-0.646$	Lemay et al[35]
BBS: Berg Balance Scale; ADL: activities of daily living; 6MWT: the 6-Minute Walk test; FTSST: Five Times Sit to Stand Test; KOOS: Knee Injury Osteoarthritis Outcome Score; SCI-FAI: Spinal Cord Injury Functional Ambulation Inventory; 10MWT: 10-Meter Walk Test		

Responsiveness/Sensitivity to Change

In a large study of 1200 Taiwanese community-dwelling, older adults, Lin et al[36] reported a small ES of the responsiveness to falls (ES=0.12), and a moderate ES for ADL decline (ES=0.42). ADL improvement on the other hand had a small ES of 0.05. French et al[37] reported similar results of a small ES of 0.33 in patients with knee osteoarthritis.

5.7: THE TIMED UP AND GO DUAL TASK

Timed Up and Go Cognitive and Timed Up and Go Manual

Purpose

The TUG dual task tests are dynamic measures for testing general mobility and risk for falls in the elderly, which includes simultaneously performing another task, either cognitive (TUG cognitive) or manual (TUG manual), during a TUG performance. Similar to the TUG, the TUG Dual Task was tested in healthy older adults and in patients with varying diagnoses to identify individuals at risk for falls.

Description

The TUG dual task has the same basic instruction as the TUG, where the participant is instructed to stand up from a standard chair, walk 3 m, turn around, walk back to the chair, and sit down. In the TUG cognitive, the participant is asked to complete the test while counting out loud or verbally counting backward by 3s from a randomly selected number between 20 and 100.[12,38] In the TUG manual, the participant is asked to walk holding a cup filled with water.[12,38]

Scoring

Time in seconds

Area of Assessment

Balance (vestibular and nonvestibular), functional mobility, and gait

ICF Domain

Activity

Time to Administer

Five minutes or less

Equipment

- Standard armchair (approximately 46 cm in height)
- Cone or other mark of distance
- Stop watch
- Cup of water

Reference Values

Only a few studies have examined the TUG dual task on healthy individuals and on different diagnostic groups (Table 5.7.1).

TABLE 5.7.1. TIMED UP AND GO DUAL TASK REFERENCE TIME IN SECONDS				
POPULATION/ DIAGNOSTIC GROUP	TUG MEAN (SD)	TUG COGNITIVE MEAN (SD)	TUG MANUAL MEAN (SD)	REFERENCES
Community- dwelling adults (age 60 to 87 years)	8.39 (1.36)	9.82 (2.39)	11.56 (2.11)	Hofheinz et al[38]
Older adults with no history of falls (mean age = 78 years, range = 65 to 85 years)	8.4 (1.7) Range = 6.4 to 12.6	9.7 (2.3) Range = 6.2 to 14.6	9.7 (1.6) Range = 6.9 to 12.6	Shumway- Cook et al[12]
Older adults with history of falls (mean age = 86.2 years, range = 76 to 95 years)	22.2(9.3) Range = 10.3 to 39	27.2(11) Range = 11 to 49.6	27.7(11.6) Range = 14 to 48	
Vestibular dysfunction	NA	12.08 (2.07)	NA	Caixeta et al[39]
Parkinson's disease	16.4 (3.8)	16.5 (3.6)* 21.5 (7.9)**	NA	Campbell et al[40]
Healthy older adults (mean age = 76.4 years, SD = 7 years)	9.85 (1.44)	10.77 (2.11)* 11.58 (2.63)**	NA	
* Low cognitive demand (repeat a sentence) ** High cognitive demand (cite days of the week in reverse) SD: standard deviation				

Minimal Detectable Change

Not established

Minimal Clinically Important Difference

Not established

Cut-Off Scores

An increase of 4.5 seconds between the TUG and TUG manual score was associated with a greater risk for falls in healthy older adults.[41] A TUG manual cut-off score of 14.5 seconds classified older adults as fallers with 90% correct prediction rate.[12] The subjects who completed the TUG cognitive in 15 seconds or longer were classified as fallers with an 87% correct prediction rate.[12]

Psychometric Properties

Reliability

In community-dwelling, older adults, test-retest reliability was excellent ($r = 0.98$).[38] Both inter-rater and intrarater reliability were also excellent in community-dwelling, older adults (interrater ICC $= 0.99$[12]; intrarater ICC $= 0.94$[38]).

Validity

In patients with Parkinson's disease, the TUG cognitive had better predictive validity of fallers (71%) than the TUG (42%). Concurrent validity with other manual and cognitive measures are listed in Table 5.7.2.

TABLE 5.7.2. CONCURRENT VALIDITY OF THE TIMED UP AND GO DUAL TASK		
POPULATION/ DIAGNOSTIC GROUP	**MEASURES THAT CORRELATE WITH TUG DUAL TASK**	**REFERENCES**
Older adults	TUG Cognitive. vs BBS, **good** correlation ($r = -0.66$)	Hofheinz et al[38]
	TUG Manual vs BBS, **good** correlation ($r = -0.72$)	
Vestibular dysfunction	TUG Cognitive vs MMSE, **low** correlation ($r_s = 0.36$)	Caixeta et al[39]
	TUG Cognitive vs Clock test, no correlation ($r_s = -0.2$)	
MMSE: Mini-Mental State Exam		

Responsiveness/Sensitivity to Change

Not established

5.8: THE 6-MINUTE WALK TEST

Link to the Instrument

http://www.cscc.unc.edu/spir/public/UNLICOMMSMWSixMinuteWalkTestFormQxQ08252011.pdf

Purpose

The original purpose of the 6-minute walk test (6MWT) was to test exercise tolerance in patients with respiratory issues and heart disease.[42] The test has since been used as a performance-based measure of functional exercise capacity in other populations including healthy, older adults.

Description

The 6MWT is a time limited test that assesses distance walked over 6 minutes within a designated test area. The testing area/walkway should be long, quiet, flat, have a hard surface, and be indoors. The American Thoracic Society suggests that the walking course be 30 m in length, marked by colored tape at every 3 m and the turnaround areas marked with a cone.[43] Participants are instructed to report if they experience shortness of breath, muscular pain, dizziness, or anginal symptoms, at which time the test is terminated. Participants are also instructed to rest whenever necessary during the test. If a participant is unable to complete the full 6 minutes of walking, then the distance covered at termination is used. Subjects can use assistive walking devices during the test.

Scoring

Distance walked, and the number and duration of rests during the 6 minutes

Area of Assessment

Submaximal aerobic capacity and gait

ICF Domain

Activity

Time to Administer

6 to 30 minutes

Equipment

- A stopwatch
- A distance measuring wheel
- A mechanical lap counter
- Two cones to mark the turnaround points
- A chair
- In patients with pulmonary and cardiac dysfunction, vital signs monitor, pulse oximeter, Borg scale, oxygen source, and access to emergency assistance are important. For this patient population, consult the American Thoracic Society guidelines.[43]

Reference Values

Reference values from 2 studies are presented in Table 5.8.1.[7,44] The generally lower scores reported by Lusardi et al[44] might be attributed to the inclusion of individuals who used assistive devices, while Steffen et al[7] included only those who ambulated independently.

TABLE 5.8.1. 6-MINUTE WALK TEST REFERENCE VALUES FOR COMMUNITY-DWELLING OLDER ADULTS IN MEATERS, MEAN (SD)

GENDER	AGE (YEARS)	STEFFEN ET AL[7] N=96	LUSARDI ET AL[44] N=76
Men	60 to 69	572 (92)	498 (0)
	70 to 79	527 (85)	475 (93)
	80 to 89	417 (73)	320 (80)
	90 to 101	———	296 (15)
Women	60 to 69	538 (92)	405 (110)
	70 to 79	471 (75)	406 (95)
	80 to 89	392 (85)	282 (123)
	90 to 101	———	261 (81)

TABLE 5.8.2. 6-MINUTE WALK TEST REFERENCE VALUES IN METERS

DIAGNOSTIC GROUP	DESCRIPTIVE STATISTICS	REFERENCES
Chronic heart failure	Mean range=310 to 427 depending on the severity of heart disease	Cahalin et al[45]
Chronic obstructive pulmonary disease	Mean=380, range=160 to 600	Casanova et al[46]
Chronic stroke	Mean=408, SD=132, range=133 to 700 (measured outdoors using GPS) Mean=413, SD=127, range=129 to 664 (measured indoors)	Wevers et al[47]
GPS: global positioning system		

Minimal Detectable Change

TABLE 5.8.3. 6-MINUTE WALK TEST MINIMAL DETECTABLE CHANGE VALUES		
POPULATION/ DIAGNOSTIC GROUP	MDC	REFERENCES
Older adults	58.21 m	Perera et al[48]
Chronic obstructive pulmonary disease	54 m	Redelmeier et al[49]
Chronic stroke	34.37 m	Eng et al[50]
	36.6 m or a 13% change	Flansbjer et al[9]
Spinal cord injury	5.8 m or a 22% change	Lam et al[51]
Parkinson's disease	82 m	Steffen and Seney[27]
Osteoarthritis	61.34 m	Kennedy et al[25]

Minimal Clinically Important Difference

TABLE 5.8.4. 6-MINUTE WALK TEST MINIMAL CLINICALLY IMPORTANT DIFFERENCE VALUES BY DIAGNOSTIC GROUP		
POPULATION/ DIAGNOSTIC GROUP	MCID	REFERENCES
Community-dwelling, older adults	50 m	Perera et al[48]
Chronic stroke	50 m	Perera et al[48]
Chronic obstructive pulmonary disease	54 m	Rasekaba et al[52]
Spinal cord injury	Walking speed of 0.10 m/s	Forrrest et al[53]

Cut-Off Scores

A distance less than 350 m is associated with increased mortality in chronic obstructive pulmonary disease (COPD), chronic heart failure, and pulmonary arterial hypertension.[52]

Psychometric Properties

Reliability

TABLE 5.8.5. 6-MINUTE WALK TEST RELIABILITY		
POPULATION/ DIAGNOSTIC GROUP	**RELIABILITY MEASURES**	**REFERENCES**
Community-dwelling adults	**Excellent** test-retest reliability (ICC = 0.95)	Steffen et al[7]
Chronic stroke	**Excellent** test-retest reliability (ICC = 0.99)	Eng et al[50]
	Excellent test-retest reliability (ICC = 0.99)	Flansbjer et al[9]
	Excellent test-retest reliability for 6MWT Outdoors (ICC = 0.96) Indoors (ICC = 0.98)	Wevers et al[47]
	Adequate intrarater reliability (ICC = 0.74) **Adequate** interrater reliability (ICC = 0.78)	Kosak and Smith[54]
Spinal cord injury	**Excellent** intrarater reliability (ICC = 0.99) **Excellent** interrater reliability (ICC = 0.99)	Scivoletto et al[55]
Alzheimer's disease	**Excellent** test-retest reliability (ICC = 0.982 to 0.987)	Ries et al[8]
	Excellent intrarater reliability (ICC = 0.76 to 0.9) **Excellent** interrater reliability (ICC = 0.97 to 0.99)	Tappen et al[56]
Osteoarthritis	**Excellent** test-retest reliability (ICC = 0.94)	Kennedy et al[25]
Traumatic brain injury	**Excellent** test-retest reliability (ICC = 0.94)	Mossberg[57]
	Excellent test-retest reliability (ICC = 0.96)	van Loo et al[58]

Validity

TABLE 5.8.6. CONCURRENT VALIDITY OF THE 6-MINUTE WALK TEST WITH OTHER FUNCTIONAL MEASURES		
POPULATION/ DIAGNOSTIC GROUP	**MEASURES THAT CORRELATE WITH 6MWT**	**REFERENCES**
Geriatrics	Chair stands, **adequate** ($r=0.67$) Standing balance, **adequate** ($r=0.52$) Gait speed **adequate** ($r=-0.73$)	Harada et al[59]
Spinal cord injury	10-Meter Walk Test, **excellent** ($r=-0.95$) TUG, **adequate** ($r=-0.88$) Walking index for SCI II, **poor** ($r=0.60$)	Lam et al[51]
	TUG, **excellent** ($r=-0.88$) 10-Meter Walk Test, **excellent** ($r=-0.95$)	van Hedel et al[28]
Chronic stroke	TUG, **excellent** ($r=-0.89$) 10-meter comfortable gait speed, **excellent** ($r=0.84$) 10-meter fast gait speed, **excellent** ($r=0.94$) Stair climbing ascend, **excellent** ($r=-0.82$) Stair climbing descend, **excellent** ($r=-0.80$)	Flansbjer et al[9]
Acute stroke	2-Minute Walk Test, **excellent** ($r=0.997$) 12-Minute Walk Test, **excellent** ($r=0.994$)	Kosak and Smith[54]
SCI: spinal cord injury		

Responsiveness/Sensitivity to Change

Based on a secondary analysis of data from a group of older adults, including patients with subacute stroke, Parera et al[48] recommended that a small meaningful change in the 6MWT is 20 m, and that a substantial meaningful change is at least 50 m.

5.9: THE 2-MINUTE WALK TEST

Link to the Instrument

http://www.rehabmeasures.org/PDF%20Library/2%20Minute%20Walk%20Test%20Instructions.pdf

Purpose

The 2-minute walk test (2MWT) is a time limited test similar to the 6MWT, except it measures a shorter time interval. This allows for testing older adults with cardiorespiratory dysfunction who are not able to perform the more rigorous 6MWT.

Description

The 2MWT measures the distance in meters walked over 2 minutes. The testing area/walkway should be long, quiet, and flat with a hard surface. The participant is instructed to report if he or she experiences shortness of breath, muscular pain, dizziness, or angina, at which time the test is terminated. The participant is also instructed to rest whenever necessary during the test. If the participant is unable to complete the full 2 minutes, then the distance covered on termination is measured. Participants can use assistive walking devices during the test, but use of devices should be kept consistent from test to test for valid comparisons.

Scoring

Distance walked and the number and duration of rests during the 2 minutes

Area of Assessment

Functional mobility, gait, and submaximal aerobic capacity

ICF Domain

Activity

Time to Administer

Five minutes or less

Equipment

- A stopwatch
- A distance measuring wheel
- A mechanical lap counter
- Two cones to mark the turnaround points
- A chair

Reference Values

TABLE 5.9.1. 2-MINUTE WALK TEST REFERENCE VALUES		
POPULATION/ DIAGNOSTIC GROUP	MEAN (SD) METERS	REFERENCES
Older adults in long-term care facilities	77.5 (25.6)	Connelly and Thomas[60]
Older adults in retirement facilities	150.4 (23.1)	
Multiple sclerosis	144 (49) Range = 92 to 630	Gijbels et al[61]
Spinal cord injury *Paraplegia* *Tetraplegia*	109.3 (48.6) Range = 11 to 212 115.9 (48) Range = 43 to 214	Lemay and Nadeau[35]
Chronic stroke	149 (48) Range = 30 to 223	Gijbels et al[62]

Minimal Detectable Change

TABLE 5.9.2. 2-MINUTE WALK TEST MINIMAL DETECTABLE CHANGE VALUES		
POPULATION/ DIAGNOSTIC GROUP	MDC (METERS)	REFERENCES
Older adults	12.2	Connelly and Thomas[60]
Chronic stroke	13.4	Hiengkaew et al[63]
Multiple sclerosis	19.21	Gijbels et al[61]
Patients with neurologic impairment	16.4	Rossier and Wade[64]
Lower extremity amputation	34.3	Resnik and Borgia[65]

Minimal Clinically Important Difference

Not established

Cut-Off Scores

Not established

Psychometric Properties

Test-Retest Reliability

The 2MWT has excellent test-retest reliability in older adults (ICC = 0.95),[60] and in patients with stroke (ICC = 0.98),[63] lower extremity amputation (ICC = 0.83),[65] neurologic impairment (ICC = 0.97),[64] and chronic obstructive pulmonary disease (COPD; $r = 0.99$).[66]

Interrater and Intrarater Reliability

In patients with acute and chronic stroke, the 2MWT demonstrated excellent interrater reliability (ICC = 0.92).[67] In patients with chronic stroke both interrater and intrarater reliability were excellent, with ICC = 0.85 for both.[63] Both interrater and intrarater reliability were excellent in patients with transtibial amputation with interrater reliability (ICCs = 0.98 to 0.99 and intrarater reliability ICCs = 0.90 to 0.96).[68] In patients with multiple sclerosis, both intrarater and interrater reliability were poor.[61]

Validity

TABLE 5.9.3. 2-MINUTE WALK TEST CONCURRENT VALIDITY WITH OTHER FUNCTIONAL MEASURES		
POPULATION/ DIAGNOSTIC GROUP	**MEASURES THAT CORRELATE WITH 2MWT**	**REFERENCES**
Older adults	BBS, **excellent** correlation ($r = 0.88$)	Connelly et al[60]
Multiple sclerosis	EDDS, **adequate** correlation ($r = 0.61$) MSWS-12, **good** correlation ($r = 0.72$)	Gijbels et al[62]
Stroke	FIM, **adequate** correlation ($r = 0.59$)	Miller et al[67]
EDDS: Kurtzke Extended Disability Status Scale; MSWS-12: The Multiple Sclerosis Walking Scale-12; FIM: Functional Independence Measure		

TABLE 5.9.4. CONSTRUCT VALIDITY OF THE 2-MINUTE WALK TEST WITH OTHER FUNCTIONAL MEASURES		
POPULATION/ DIAGNOSTIC GROUP	**MEASURES THAT CORRELATE WITH 2MWT**	**REFERENCES**
Older adults	6MWT, **excellent** correlation ($r=0.93$) TUG, **excellent** correlation ($r=-0.87$)	Connelly et al[60]
Inpatient older adults ***n=52; mean age=79.9 years (SD=7.7)***	FIM, **adequate** correlation ($r=0.47$ to 0.59) TUG, **excellent** correlation ($r=0.81$ to 0.68) Modified Barthel index, **adequate** correlation ($r=0.35$ to 0.42) FRT, **adequate** correlation ($r=0.41$ to 0.51)	Brooks et al[69]
Stroke	6MWT, **excellent** correlation ($r=0.997$)	Kosak and Smith[70]
Chronic obstructive pulmonary disease	6MWT, **excellent** correlation ($r=0.937$) VO2max, **adequate** correlation ($r=0.454$) VO2max/kg, **adequate** correlation ($r=0.555$)	Leung et al[66]
Lower extremity amputation ***Mean age=45 years (SD=7)***	Locomotors capabilities index, **excellent** correlation ($r=0.71$; $P<0.01$)	Salavati et al[71]
Multiple sclerosis	6MWT, **excellent** correlation ($r=0.97$; $P<0.01$)	Gijbels et al[62]
Spinal cord injury	10MWT ($r=0.932$; $P<0.01$) TUG ($r=0.623$; $P<0.01$) BBS ($r=0.781$; $P<0.01$)	Lemay and Nadeau[35]
FRT: Functional Reach Test; VO2max: maximum oxygen consumption		

Responsiveness/Sensitivity to Change

The 2MWT has been shown to be responsive to change in older adults,[72] in patients with lower extremity amputation,[73] stroke,[70] COPD,[66] multiple sclerosis,[74] and in patients after coronary artery bypass graft surgery.[75] Leung et al[66] reported significant improvement after 5 weeks of pulmonary rehabilitation in patients with COPD with an increase of 17.2 m (SD = 13.8) on the 2MWT with an ES of 0.61.

5.10: THE DYNAMIC GAIT INDEX

Link to the Instrument

http://www.dartmouth-hitchcock.org/dhmc-internet-upload/file_collection/gait_0109.pdf

Purpose

The Dynamic Gait Index (DGI) assesses the ability of the individual to maintain walking balance while responding to different task demands, during various dynamic conditions. The DGI was originally developed to assess the likelihood of falling in community-dwelling, older adults.[76,77]

Description

The DGI consists of 8 walking tasks with varying demands, including (1) walking on a level surface, (2) walking and changing speed, (3 and 4) walking while turning the head in a horizontal and vertical direction, (5) maintaining walking balance during rapid directional changes, (6 and 7) walking and stepping over and around an obstacle, and (8) climbing stairs. The highest possible score is 24 points.

Scoring

The score for each of the 8 items is based on a 4-point scale (0 to 3), where 3 = no dysfunction, 2 = minimal impairment, 1 = moderate impairment, and 0 = severe impairment.

Area of Assessment

Gait, balance (vestibular and nonvestibular), and functional mobility

ICF Domain

Activity

Time to Administer

Ten minutes or less

Equipment

- A 6-meter walkway
- Shoe box
- Two identical obstacles
- Stairs

Reference Values

Vereek et al[78] reported DGI reference values for 318 asymptomatic adults (age 20 and older), who did not report a fall in the previous 6 months (Table 5.10.1). DGI scores showed a marked decline in the eighth decade (median score: 22, range = 13 to 24), and to a lesser extent in the seventh decade (median score: 23.2, range = 21 to 24).[78]

TABLE 5.10.1. DYNAMIC GAIT INDEX REFERENCE VALUES FOR ADULTS[78]				
DECADE	N	DGI, MEAN	SD	RANGE
3	74	24	0.2	23 to 24
4	45	24	0.2	23 to 24
5	41	23.9	0.4	22 to 24
6	39	23.9	0.4	22 to 24
7	60	23.2	0.9	21 to 24
8	59	22	2	13 to 24

Minimal Detectable Change

TABLE 5.10.2. DYNAMIC GAIT INDEX MINIMAL DETECTABLE CHANGE VALUES		
POPULATION/ DIAGNOSTIC GROUP	MDC	REFERENCES
Community-dwelling, older adults	2.9 points	Romero et al[79]
Multiple sclerosis	4.19 to 5.54 points*	Cattaneo et al[80]
Chronic stroke	2.6 points*	Jonsdottir and Cattaneo[81]
Stroke	4 points Percent change = 16.6%	Lin et al[82]
Parkinson's disease	2.9 points MDC = 13.3%	Huang et al[83]
Vestibular disorders	3.2 points*	Hall and Herdman[84]
*MDCs are calculated from standard error of measurement by the reviewers of the Rehabilitation Measures Database: www.rehabmeasures.org.		

Minimal Clinically Important Difference

Through a secondary analysis of data from a randomized controlled trial, Pardasaney et al[85] reported an MCID of 1.90 points for a group of older adults (older than 65 years, 28% were 80 years of age or older). When subjects were divided according to their DGI scores, the MCID was 1.80 points for subjects with DGI scores < 21/24 and 0.60 for subjects with DGI scores > 21/24.[85]

Cut-Off Scores

Several studies have reported that the DGI has a ceiling effect in high-functioning, community-dwelling, older adults.[78,86,87]

TABLE 5.10.3. DYNAMIC GAIT INDEX MINIMAL DETECTABLE CHANGE VALUES		
POPULATION/ DIAGNOSTIC GROUP	CUT-OFF SCORE	REFERENCES
Community-dwelling adults	< 19 (sensitivity 59%; specificity 64%)	Shumway-Cook et al[76]
	< 19 (sensitivity 67%; specificity 86%)	Wrisley and Kumar[31]
Parkinson's disease	< 19 (sensitivity 64%; specificity 85%)	Dibble et al[22]
	< 18.5 (sensitivity 68%; specificity 78%)	Landers et al[88]
Multiple sclerosis	< 12 (sensitivity 45%; specificity 80%)	Cattaneo et al[89]
Vestibular disorders	< 19/24 are 2.58 times more likely to have reported a fall in the previous 6 months.	Whitney et al[90]

Psychometric Properties

Test-Retest Reliability

The DGI had excellent test-retest reliability for the total score in patients with Parkinson's disease (ICC = 0.84),[83] multiple sclerosis (ICC = 0.85),[80] vestibular disorders (ICC = 0.86),[80] and stroke (ICC = 0.94).[82]

Interrater and Intrarater Reliability

Using the Danish version of the DGI, Jonsson et al[91] reported excellent interrater and intrarater reliability, when evaluating hospitalized and community-dwelling, older adults with balance impairment. The interrater ICC for the community-dwelling group was 0.82, while the intrarater ICC was 0.90 for the hospital group; the ICCs were 0.92 and 0.90 respectively.[91] The DGI had excellent interrater reliability when used with patients with multiple sclerosis (ICC = 0.98)[92] and patients with stroke (ICC = 0.96).[81] However, the DGI had only moderate interrater reliability (overall kappa = 0.64) when used in people with vestibular disorders.[93] The DGI intrarater reliability was excellent in patients with multiple sclerosis with ICCs ranging from 0.760 to 0.98.[92]

Concurrent Validity

TABLE 5.10.4. CONCURRENT VALIDITY OF THE DYNAMIC GAIT INDEX WITH OTHER FUNCTIONAL MEASURES		
POPULATION/ DIAGNOSTIC GROUP	**MEASURES THAT CORRELATE WITH DGI**	**REFERENCES**
Community-dwelling, older adults	Balance self-perceptions test, **excellent** ($r=0.76$) BBS, **excellent** ($r=0.67$) Assistive devices history, **adequate** ($r=-0.44$) History of imbalance, **adequate** ($r=-0.46$)	Shumway-Cook et al[76]
Parkinson's disease	UPDRS-motor subscale scores, **adequate** ($r=-0.567$) History of falls, **excellent** ($r=0.643$)	Cakit et al[94]
Multiple sclerosis	BBS, **excellent** ($r_s=0.78$) TUG, **excellent** ($r_s=-0.80$) ABC, **adequate** ($r_s=-0.5$) DHI, **poor** ($r_s=-0.39$)	Cattaneo et al[89] Cattaneo et al[80]
Vestibular disorders	BBS, **excellent** ($r=-0.71$)	Whitney et al[90]
Acute stroke ***(3-time assessment: week 1, 2 months, and 5 months of therapy)***	DGI-4 and FGA, **excellent** ($r_s>0.91$) 10MWT, **excellent** ($r_s=0.61$ to 0.87)	Lin et al[82]
Chronic stroke	BBS, **excellent** ($r=0.83$) ABC, **excellent** ($r=0.68$)	Jonsdottir and Cattaneo[81]
UPDRS-motor: Unified Parkinson's Disease Rating Scale; ABC: Activities-Specific Balance Confidence Scale; DHI: Dizziness Handicap Inventory; DGI-4: 4-Item Dynamic Gait Index; FGA: Functional Gait Assessment		

Responsiveness/Sensitivity to Change

The DGI had poor responsiveness in community-dwelling, older adults after 16 weeks of exercise, with a small ES of 0.27.[85] For participants with low baseline scores (< 21/24) the ES was 0.64.[85] Moderate responsiveness was reported in patients with acute and chronic stroke after 2 months of rehabilitation with an ES of 0.56, which increased to 0.62 at 5 months.[82]

5.11: VARIATIONS OF THE DYNAMIC GAIT INDEX

The 4-Item Dynamic Gait Index

Purpose

The purpose of the DGI-4 is similar to the original DGI as it also assesses the ability of the individual to maintain walking balance while responding to different task demands. It includes only 4 of the 8 items of the original DGI, it is faster to perform and requires no equipment.[95]

Description

The DGI-4 consists of 4 walking tasks on a level surface: (1) walking on a level surface, (2) walking and changing gait speed, (3) walking while turning the head in a horizontal direction, and (4) walking while turning the head in a vertical direction. The highest possible score is 12 points.

Scoring

The score for each of the 4 items is based on a 4-point scale (0 to 3), where 3 = no gait dysfunction, 2 = minimal impairment, 1 = moderate impairment, and 0 = severe impairment.

Area of Assessment

Gait, balance (vestibular and nonvestibular), and functional mobility

ICF Domain

Activity

Time to Administer

Five minutes or less

Equipment

None

Reference Values

In subjects with balance and vestibular disorders (n = 123), those who did not report a fall had significantly higher DGI-4 total scores (mean = 9.0) compared to those subjects who reported falls in the previous 6 months (mean = 7.1).[95]

Cut-Off Scores

A score less than 12 out of 12 identifies individuals with balance deficits.[95] A score of less than 10 out of 12 on the DGI-4 indicates a risk for falls,[95] while a score of 9 or less has 56% sensitivity and 62% specificity in identifying fallers and nonfallers.[95]

Psychometric Properties

The psychometric properties of the DGI-4 were comparable or superior to those of the original 8-item DGI.[95] The DGI-4 also correlates with Falls Efficacy Scale-International (FES-I) in people with vestibular disorders (r_s = -.055).[96]

The Modified Dynamic Gait Index

Link to the Instrument

This form is available in the appendix of the original article:

Shumway-Cook A, Taylor CS, Matsuda PN, Studer MT, Whetten BK. Expanding the scoring system for the Dynamic Gait Index. *Phys Ther.* 2013;93(11):1493-1506.

Purpose

The Modified Dynamic Gait Index (mDGI) expands the original 8-Item DGI providing a greater range of possible scores. In addition to DGI scoring, it scores the level of assistance (LOA), gait pattern (GP), and time for each of the 8 items.[97] The test has 4 environmental dimensions: temporal, postural, terrain, and density.

Description

The same 8-Item DGI tasks were retained for the mDGI, however, minor modifications were implemented to clarify the procedure and facilitate using a new scoring system. These modifications are:

- A 6.1-meter walkway was used for all tasks.
- The change of pace task includes an acceleration phase ("walk as quickly as you safely can"), but no deceleration was imposed for any of the tasks.
- The dimensions of the obstacles are specified as 76 cm long, 12 cm wide, and 5 cm thick. The first obstacle is placed 2.4 m (8 ft) from the starting point, with the 12-cm side flat on the floor. The second obstacle is placed with the 12-cm side up and placed 2.4 m past the first obstacle (about 4.9 m [16 ft] from the start).
- The pivot turn task includes a turn halfway through the course with a return to the starting position, rather than a stop.
- The stairs task measures performance only while ascending but not descending.

Scoring

While scoring for the 8-Item DGI is limited to a single score from 0 to 3 for each item, the mDGI gives 3 separate scores for each item as follows:

- **Time:** time to complete each task performed over a 6.1-m course—converted to 4-level scale (varies per question)
- **LOA:** 3-level scale
  - 2 = no assistance
  - 1 = uses an assistive device (not including orthosis/braces)
  - 0 = requires the physical assistance of another person includes contact guard
- **GP:** 4-level scale (varies per question)
  - 3 = normal: no evidence for imbalance
  - 2 = mild impairment: mild gait deviations
  - 1 = moderate impairment: moderate gait deviations, evidence of imbalance but recovers independently
  - 0 = severe impairment: severe gait deviations, or loses balance and unable to recover independently

The total mDGI score = 0 to 64 points
- Total time facet points = 0 to 24 points
- Total LOA facet points = 0 to 16 points
- Total GP facet points = 0 to 24 points

Area of Assessment

Gait, balance (vestibular and nonvestibular), and functional mobility

ICF Domain

Activity

Time to Administer

Ten minutes or less

Equipment

- 6.1-m (20-ft) walkway
- Measuring tape
- Stopwatch
- Tape for marking start point, 10-ft and 20-ft points along the walkway
- Two semirigid foam rectangle obstacles (76 cm long, 12 cm diameter, 5 cm thick)

Reference Values

TABLE 5.11.1. MODIFIED DYNAMIC GAIT INDEX REFERENCE VALUES[97]						
MEASURE	**MOBILITY IMPAIRED GROUP**			**CONTROL GROUP**		
	n	*X*	*SD*	*n*	*X*	*SD*
mDGI total score	698	40.74	14.53	117	53.16	14.01
FACETS OF PERFORMANCE SCORES						
Time score	701	12.30	6.49	117	18.44	6.34
Gait pattern score	702	15.94	4.78	118	20.10	5.16
Level of assistance score	705	12.52	5.08	118	14.48	3.38
TASK SCORES						
Usual pace	857	5.55	1.73	138	6.84	1.59
Change pace	856	5.38	1.88	138	6.83	1.61
Horizontal head turns	856	4.95	1.91	138	6.46	1.93
Vertical head turns	857	5.08	1.92	138	6.46	2.08
Pivot turn	857	5.22	1.89	138	6.53	1.89
Stepping over obstacles	854	5.03	2.23	136	6.48	2.33
Stepping around obstacles	856	5.53	1.80	138	6.92	1.50
Stairs	702	4.75	2.19	118	6.31	2.36

Minimal Detectable Change

The mDGI, 95% MDC for patients in 5 diagnostic groups (stroke, vestibular dysfunction, traumatic brain injury, gait abnormality, and Parkinson's disease), was 7.0 for the total score (3.1 for time, 4.0 for GP, and 2.4 for LOA).[98] In the control group with no neurologic disorder the MDC was 5.5 for the total score (2.5 for time, 3.2 for GP, and 1.9 for LOA).[98]

Psychometric Properties

Test-retest of the mDGI is excellent for time ($r = 0.91$), GP ($r = 0.91$), and LOA ($r = 0.87$).[97] Interrater reliability for level of assistance had strong agreement (kappa = 0.84 to 1.00), for gait pattern it was moderate to strong (kappa = 0.59 to 0.88), and for time it was strong (kappa = 0.90 to 0.98).[97]

The Functional Gait Assessment

Link to the Instrument

This form is available in the appendix of the original article:
Wrisley DM, Marchetti GF, Kuharsky DK, Whitney SL. Reliability, internal consistency, and validity of data obtained with the functional gait assessment. *Phys Ther.* 2004;84(10):906-918.

Purpose

The FGA is an expansion of the DGI assessing postural stability during various walking tasks. The FGA provides a higher degree of difficulty in testing in order to reduce the ceiling effect of the DGI.

Description

The test is composed of 10 items which include 7 of the 8 items from the original DGI (eliminated ambulation around obstacles), and added 3 more challenging new items including walking with a narrow base of support, walking backwards, and walking with eyes closed. Assessment may be performed with or without an assistive device.

Scoring

Each item is scored on a 4-point scale from 0 to 3, with
- 0 = severe impairment
- 1 = moderate impairment
- 2 = mild impairment
- 3 = normal ambulation
Highest total score = 30

Area of Assessment

Gait, balance (vestibular and nonvestibular), and functional mobility

ICF Domain

Activity

Time to Administer

Ten minutes or less

Equipment

- Stopwatch
- Marked walking area: Length = 6.1 m (20 feet); width 30.5 cm (12 inches)
- Obstacle height of 2.86 cm (9 inches) using at least 2 stacked shoe boxes
- Set of steps with railings

Reference Values

TABLE 5.11.2. FUNCTIONAL GAIT ASSESSMENT REFERENCE VALUES FOR OLDER ADULTS[99]				
AGE (YEARS)	N	MEAN	SD	95% CI
40 to 49	27	28.9	1.5	28.3 to 29.5
50 to 59	33	28.4	1.6	27.9 to 29.0
60 to 69	63	27.1	2.3	26.5 to 27.7
70 to 79	44	24.9	3.6	23.9 to 26.0
80 to 89	33	20.8	4.7	19.2 to 22.6
Total	200	26.1	4	25.5 to 26.6
CI: confidence interval				

Minimal Detectable Change

Measurement of FGA scores in patients with stroke after 5 months of outpatient rehabilitation demonstrated an average increase of 4.2 points (5 points clinically) that can be interpreted as a real change with 95% confidence.[90]

Minimal Clinically Important Difference

In a retrospective analysis of patients with vestibular disorders, Marchetti et al[100] demonstrated that the amount of pre- to posttreatment change exceeding chance variation was estimated to be 6 points. This change was significantly associated with improvement in self-reported disability as measured by the ABC and the DHI.

Cut-Off Scores

A score of 22/30 provided 100% sensitivity and 72% specificity in predicting fallers and nonfallers in community-dwelling, older adults.[31]

Psychometric Properties

Reliability

TABLE 5.11.3. RELIABILITY OF THE FUNCTIONAL GAIT ASSESSMENT		
POPULATION/ DIAGNOSTIC GROUP	CORRELATION COEFFICIENTS	REFERENCES
Older adults	Interrater reliability, **excellent** (ICC = 0.93)	Walker et al[99]
Vestibular disorders	Interrater, **excellent** (ICC = 0.84) Intrarater (ICC = 0.83)	Wrisley et al[31]
Parkinson's disease	Test-retest administered by physical therapist, **excellent** (ICC = 0.91) Test-retest administered by student, **excellent** (ICC = 0.80) Interrater reliability, **excellent** (ICC = 0.93)	Leddy et al[101]
Acute and chronic stroke	Test-retest reliability, **excellent** (ICC = 0.95)	Lin et al[90]
Subacute stroke	Interrater reliability, **excellent** (ICC = 0.94) Intrarater reliability, **excellent** (ICC = 0.97)	Thieme et al[102]

Validity

TABLE 5.11.4. CONCURRENT VALIDITY OF THE FUNCTIONAL GAIT ASSESSMENT WITH OTHER FUNCTIONAL MEASURES		
POPULATION/ DIAGNOSTIC GROUP	**MEASURES THAT CORRELATE WITH THE FUNCTIONAL GAIT ASSESSMENT**	**REFERENCES**
Community- dwelling adults	BBS, **excellent** ($r=0.84$) TUG test, **excellent** ($r=0.84$) ABC, **adequate** ($r=0.53$)	Wrisley et al[31]
Parkinson's disease	BBS, **excellent** ($r=0.77$) PDQ-39 mobility subsection, **excellent** ($r=-0.66$) Postural instability gait disorder score, **excellent** ($r=-0.689$) total score, **adequate** ($r=-0.57$) Bradykinesia composite score, **adequate** ($r=-0.55$) Freezing of gait score, **adequate** ($r=-0.54$) Functional reach, **adequate** ($r=0.52$) 9-Hole Peg Test, **adequate** ($r=-0.52$)	Ellis et al[103]
Stroke	10MWT and PASS, **excellent** ($r=-0.66$ to 0.83) Functional Ambulatory Category, **excellent** ($r=0.83$) Gait speed, **excellent** ($r=0.82$) BBS, **excellent** ($r=0.93$) Rivermead Mobility Index, **excellent** ($r=0.85$) Barthel Index, **excellent** ($r=0.71$)	Thieme et al[102]
Vestibular disorders	Perception Dizziness Symptoms, **excellent** ($r=-0.70$) Dizziness Handicap Inventory, **excellent** ($r=-0.64$) ABC, **excellent** ($r=0.64$) Number of falls in previous 4 weeks, **excellent** ($r=-0.66$) DGI, **excellent** ($r=0.80$) TUG, **adequate** ($r=-0.50$)	Wrisley et al[31]
PDQ-39: Parkinson's Disease Questionnaire-39; PASS: Postural Assessment Scale for Stroke Patients		

Responsiveness/Sensitivity to Change

The FGA displayed moderate responsiveness in detecting change in patients with acute and chronic stroke at 2 and 5 months after rehabilitation. The ES was 0.50 at 2 months and 0.54 at 5 months.[90]

5.12: The 360° Turn Test

Purpose

The 360° Turn Test assesses dynamic balance. The participant turns in a complete circle, 360 degrees (taking steps), while the examiner records the time (in seconds) and/or the number of steps. The turn can be made in either direction.[104]

Description

The participant stands at a specific spot, marked on the floor with a piece of masking tape, in a comfortable posture with arms by the sides, feet shoulder-width apart, and facing the examiner. The examiner asks the participant to turn in a circle, while taking steps, in either direction. Timing starts from the word "go" and stops when the participant is back to the starting position facing the examiner. The participant performs 2 consecutive trials in the same direction, and the examiner records the average of the 2 trials.

Scoring

Time (seconds) or number of steps

Area of Assessment

Balance and gait

ICF Domain

Activity

Time to Administer

Five minutes or less

Equipment

- Stop watch
- Masking tape

Reference Values

TABLE 5.12.1. 360° TURN TEST REFERENCE VALUES FOR COMMUNITY-DWELLING, OLDER ADULTS[105]		
GROUPS	MEAN (SECONDS)	STANDARD DEVIATION
Nonfall group n=372, age 71 (9.3) years	2.2	0.9
Fall group n=139, age 75 (11) years	2.7	1.5

TABLE 5.12.2. 360° TURN TEST REFERENCE VALUES FOR PATIENTS WITH PARKINSON'S DISEASE			
HOEHN AND YAHR STAGE	**360° TURN TIME (SECONDS)**	**360° NUMBER OF STEPS**	**REFERENCES**
2 (n=8) 3 (n=7)	Mean=6.0 (2.5) Range=3.8 to 15.9	Mean=9.5 (2.9) Range=5.5 to 18.5	Schenkman et al[106]
2 to 3 n=15	"OFF" (levodopa) State, Mean=5.3 (1.6) "ON" (levodopa) State, Mean=5.1 (1.9)	NA	Franzen et al[107]
1 to 1.5	Mean=3.33 (0.98)	6.33 (0.93)	Schenkman et al[108]
2	Mean=3.91 (1.37)	7.55 (1.96)	
2.5	Mean=4.81 (1.58)	8.66 (2.66)	
3	Mean=7.34 (3.60)	11.04 (3.61)	
n total=150			

Minimal Detectable Change

Shiu et al[109] demonstrated an MDC of 0.76 seconds in patients with chronic stroke when turning toward the affected side, and 1.22 seconds for the same patients turning toward the unaffected side.

Minimal Clinically Important Difference

Not established

Cut-Off Scores

Time >3.8 seconds is associated with increased ADL dependence in community-dwelling, older adults (age ≥70 years).[104]

Psychometric Properties

Reliability

TABLE 5.12.3. RELIABILITY OF THE 360° TURN TEST			
TYPE OF RELIABILITY	**GROUP**	**CORRELATION COEFFICIENTS**	**REFERENCES**
Test-retest	Community-dwelling, older adults (n = 199, age ≥55 years)	360° Turn Test (steps), **excellent** (ICC = 0.92)	Tager et al[110]
	Parkinson's disease	360° Turn Test (sec), **excellent** (ICC = 0.77) 360° Turn Test (steps), **excellent** (ICC = 0.80)	Schenkman et al[106]
	Chronic stroke (n = 72)	360° Turn Test (sec), **excellent** (ICC = 0.94; affected side) (ICC = 0.824; unaffected side)	Shu[109]
Intrarater	History of falls and a variety of diagnoses (n = 38, mean age 73 years)	360° Turn item on the BBS: Time 1, **excellent** (ICC = 0.89) Time 2, **excellent** (ICC = 0.94)	Berg[111]
	Chronic stroke (n = 72)	360° Turn Test (sec) Time 1, **excellent** (ICC = 0.952; affected side) Time 2, **excellent** (ICC = 0.927; unaffected side)	Shu[109]
Interrater	Chronic stroke (n = 72)	360° Turn Test (sec), **excellent** (ICC = 0.991; affected side), **excellent** (ICC = 0.993; unaffected side)	Shu[109]

TABLE 5.12.4. VALIDITY OF THE 360° TURN TEST		
POPULATION/ DIAGNOSTIC GROUP	MEASURES THAT CORRELATE WITH 360° TURN TEST	REFERENCES
Community-dwelling, older adults *n = 195, mean age = 80.9 (SD = 5.9)*	Tandem Stance Test, **adequate** (r = 0.46) Walking speed, **excellent** (r = 0.70) Timed chair rise(s), **poor** (r = 0.26)	Shubert et al[112]
Older adults *n = 10, mean age = 63.06 (SD = 6.3)*	180° Turn Test (sec), **excellent** (r = 0.67) 180° Turn Test (steps), **excellent** (r = 0.76)	Dite et al[113]
Parkinson's disease *n = 34, Hoen and Yahr Stage mean = 2.07 (SD = 0.79)*	CS-PFP (sec), **adequate** (r = -0.53) CS-PFP (steps), **adequate** (r = -0.54)	Schenkman et al[106]
Chronic stroke *(n = 72)*	BBS, **excellent** (r_s = -0.758) 10MWT, **excellent** (r = 0.662) TUG, **excellent** (r_s = -0.759)	Shu[109]
CS-PFP: Continuous Scale-Physical Functional Performance		

Responsiveness/Sensitivity to Change

Gill et al[114] studied the association between change in physical performance and the onset of ADL dependence in a group of older adults at baseline and 1 year later. ADL dependence developed in 12% of the group (n = 96) at the 1-year follow-up. Those individuals took longer to complete the 360° Turn Test (mean = 2.3 [8.80] sec) compared to those who remained independent (mean = 0.37 [3.57] sec).[114]

5.13: THE FOUR SQUARE STEP TEST

Link to Instrument

http://www.rehabmeasures.org/PDF%20Library/Four%20Step%20Square%20Test%20Instructions.pdf

Purpose

The Four Square Step Test (FSST) assesses dynamic balance. It is a timed stepping test that challenges the ability to change the base of support by shifting weight from one foot to the other, while stepping over low objects, and changing direction in a structured format in forward, lateral, and backward directions.

Description

A plus sign-shaped grid is placed on the floor using 4 canes or plastic pipes to create four quadrants. The participant begins standing in the rear-left quadrant (square 1), steps forward over the first bar to stand in square 2, steps to the right to stand in the right-front quadrant (square 3), steps backward to the right-rear quadrant (square 4), and then steps to the left to stand in the starting location (square 1).

The participant then reverses direction (counterclockwise), stepping through each quadrant in the same manner until he or she stands again in the rear-left quadrant. Participant instructions are as follows: "Try to complete the sequence as fast as possible without touching the sticks. Both feet must make contact with the floor in each square. If possible, face forward during the entire sequence."

Scoring

After a practice trial, the participant performs 2 trials and the better (shorter) time in seconds is recorded. Timing starts when the first foot touches square 2 and ends when the last foot touches square 1.

Area of Assessment

Balance and daily activities that require stepping

ICF Domain

Activity

Time to Administer

Five minutes

Equipment

- A stopwatch
- Four canes, bars, or pipes

Reference Values

TABLE 5.13.1. FOUR SQUARE STEP TEST REFERENCE VALUES		
POPULATION/ DIAGNOSTIC GROUP	TIME (SECONDS) MEAN (SD)	REFERENCES
Older adults with transtibial amputation	Recurrent Falls: 32.6 (10.1) No Recurrent Falls: 17.6 (8.3)	Dite et al[115]
Acute stroke	20.8 (15.0) Range = 6.1 to 60.1	Blennerhassett and Jayalath[116]
Parkinson's disease	On medication: 9.6 Range = 8.73 to 10.62 Off medication: 11.02 Range = 9.42 to 12.56	Duncan and Earhart et al[117]

Minimal Detectable Change

Not established

Minimal Clinically Important Difference

Not established

Cut-Off Scores

TABLE 5.13.2. FOUR SQUARE STEP TEST CUT-OFF SCORES INDICATING RISK OF FALLS		
POPULATION/ DIAGNOSTIC GROUP	**CUT-OFF SCORE (SECONDS)**	**REFERENCES**
Older adults	> 15	Dite and Temple[115]
Acute stroke	> 15	Blennerhassett and Jaylath[116]
Parkinson's disease	> 9.68	Duncan and Earhart et al[117]
Transtibial amputation	> 24	Dite et al[20]
Vestibular disorders	> 12	Whitney et al[118]

Psychometric Properties

Reliability

TABLE 5.13.3. RELIABILITY OF THE FOUR SQUARE STEP TEST		
POPULATION/ DIAGNOSTIC GROUP	**CORRELATION COEFFICIENTS**	**REFERENCES**
Older adults	Test-retest, **excellent** (ICC = 0.98) Interrater reliability, **excellent** (ICC = 0.99)	Dite and Temple[115]
Vestibular disorders	Test-retest, **excellent** (ICC = 0.93)	Whitney et al[118]
Parkinson's disease	On medication: test-retest, **excellent** (ICC = 0.78) Off medication: test-retest, **excellent** (ICC = 0.90) Interrater reliability, **excellent** (ICC = 0.99)	Duncan and Earhart et al[117]

Validity

TABLE 5.13.4. CONCURRENT VALIDITY OF THE FOUR SQUARE STEP TEST WITH OTHER FUNCTIONAL MEASURES		
POPULATION/ DIAGNOSTIC GROUP	**MEASURES THAT CORRELATE WITH FSST**	**REFERENCES**
Older adults	Step Test, **excellent** ($r=-0.83$) TUG test, **excellent** ($r=0.88$) FRT, **fair** ($r=-0.47$)	Dite and Temple[115]
Parkinson's disease	MDS-UPDRS Scale III, **good** ($r_s=0.61$) Mini Best ($r=-0.65$) 5 Times to Sit to Stand ($r_s=0.58$) 6MWT ($r_s=-0.52$) 9-Hole Peg Test, **good** ($r_s=0.65$) Freezing of Gait Questionnaire ($r_s=0.44$)	Duncan and Earhart et al[117]
Vestibular disorders	TUG test, **adequate** ($r=0.69$) Gait Speed, **adequate** ($r=0.65$) DGI, **adequate** ($r=-0.51$) Dizziness Handicap Inventory, **poor** ($r=-0.13$) ABC, **poor** ($r=-0.12$)	Whitney et al[118]
Acute stroke	Step test: right and left stance, **excellent** ($r_s=0.86$)	Blennerhassett and Jayalath[116]
MDS-UPDRS: Movement Disorder Society Unified Parkinson's Disease Rating Scale		

Responsiveness/Sensitivity to Change

After 4 weeks of rehabilitation, patients with stroke, who could walk at least 50 m with minimal assistance at baseline, showed an ES of 0.33.[116]

5.14: The Functional Ambulation Classification

Link to Instrument

http://www.rehabmeasures.org/PDF%20Library/Functional%20Ambulation%20Category%20Test%20Instructions.pdf

Purpose

The Functional Ambulation Classification (FAC) is a walking test that classifies subjects into 6 functional categories based on the need for personal assistance, regardless of the use of a walking assistive device. It was originally designed for patients after a stroke.[119,120]

Description

The evaluator briefly observes the subject while walking and provides a rating from 0 to 5. A score of 0 indicates that the participant is a nonfunctional ambulator (cannot walk), while a score of 5 describes an independent ambulator who can walk independently on any surface.[119]

Scoring

- 0: Participant cannot walk, or needs help from 2 or more persons
- 1: Participant needs firm continuous support from one person who helps carry participant's weight and assists with balance
- 2: Participant needs continuous or intermittent support of one person to help with balance and coordination
- 3: Participant requires verbal supervision or stand-by help from one person without physical contact
- 4: Participant can walk independently on level ground, but requires help on stairs, slopes, or uneven surfaces
- 5: Participant can walk independently

Area of Assessment

Gait and functional mobility

ICF Domain

Activity

Time to Administer

Two minutes or less

Equipment

None

Reference Values

Kollen et al[121] scored the FAC and gait speed on patients with acute stroke, and obtained weekly measurements from week 4 to week 26 after the stroke. Only data of patients with FAC scores of 3 to 5 were included because these patients required no assistance. Patients who were evaluated as having 3 on the FAC had a gait speed between 0.19 to 0.45 m/s, a score of 4 corresponded to a gait speed between 0.48 to 0.90 m/s, while a score of 5 matched a gait speed of 0.92 to 1.11 m/s.[121]

TABLE 5.14.1. FUNCTIONAL AMBULATION CLASSIFICATION SCORES AND CORRESPONDING GAIT SPEED IN PATIENTS WITH ACUTE STROKE[121]															
FAC SCORE	NUMBER OF SUBJECTS	WALKING SPEED (M/S) BY NUMBER OF WEEKS AFTER THE STROKE													
		4	5	6	7	8	9	10	12	14	16	18	20	26
3	11	0.45	0.43	0.37	0.45	0.33	0.39	0.38	0.35	0.33	0.29	0.30	0.30	0.19
4	12	0.73	0.90	0.80	0.63	0.65	0.64	0.58	0.57	0.50	0.50	0.49	0.48	0.48
5	2	1.08	0.92	1.04	1.04	1.06	1.02	1.11	1.07	1.06	1.04	1.00	1.02	0.92

Minimal Detectable Change

Not established

Minimal Clinically Important Difference

Not established

Cut-Off Scores

A cut-off score of 4 or more predicted community ambulators, 6 months after a stroke, with 100% sensitivity and 78% specificity.[122]

Psychometric Properties

Reliability

Mehrholz et al[122] reported excellent test-retest reliability (Kappa = 0.95), as well as excellent interrater reliability (Kappa = 0.95) in 55 patients between 30 and 60 days after the first stroke.

TABLE 5.14.2. CONCURRENT VALIDITY OF THE FUNCTIONAL AMBULATION CLASSIFICATION WITH OTHER FUNCTIONAL MEASURES		
DIAGNOSTIC GROUP	**MEASURES THAT CORRELATE WITH THE FAC**	**REFERENCES**
Chronic stroke	Walking velocity, **good** ($r=0.67$) Cadence, **good** ($r=0.62$)	Holden et al[123]
Acute stroke	RMI, **good** ($r_s=0.686$) 6MWT, **excellent** ($r_s=0.949$) Walking velocity, **excellent** ($r_s=0.952$) Step length, **excellent** ($r_s=0.952$)	Mehrholz et al[122]
RMI: Rivermead Mobility Index		

Responsiveness/Sensitivity to Change

FAC scores changed significantly with an SRM of 1.016 within the first 2 weeks of a 6-month stroke rehabilitation program.[121] FAC scores continued to significantly increase with an SRM of 0.699 at the end of the program which suggested that the FAC can be used to measure change in gait performance outcomes in patients after stroke.[121]

Kollen et al[121] demonstrated decreased responsiveness of the FAC in stroke patients at lower levels of function. They also cautioned that a change in walking speed over time, could shift the FAC appraisal to a lower score at a higher speed.[121]

5.15: THE MODIFIED GAIT ABNORMALITY RATING SCALE

Link to Instrument

http://mobile-pt.com/files/GAIT_ABNOMALITY_RATING_SCALE.pdf

Purpose

The Modified Gait Abnormality Rating Scale (GARS-M) was developed to estimate fall risk in community-dwelling and frail elderly adults.[124] The GARS-M is a shorter (7-item) version of the original 16-item Gait Abnormality Rating Scale (GARS), which was developed for elderly individuals residing in nursing homes.[125] The items removed from the original GARS were either redundant or difficult to visually rate, had low interrater reliability, or were not good differentiators between fallers and nonfallers.[124] Gait variability, a unique aspect of the GARS-M, has been linked to increased fall risk in older adults.[126]

Description

The participant is videotaped while walking at a self-selected pace on a level surface of about 8 m, then he or she turns and walks back to the original point. The video recorded gait is then examined and each of 7 items is scored on a 4 point scale (0 to 3), where 0 = normal, 1 = mildly impaired, 2 = moderately impaired, and 3 = severely impaired. The total score ranges from 0 to 21, with a higher score indicating greater impairment and fall risk.

Scoring

The following 7 items of the subjects' gait are evaluated during videotape playback in slow motion: (1) gait variability, (2) guardedness, (3) staggering, (4) Initial Contact, (5) hip range of motion, (6) shoulder extension, and (7) arm-heel strike synchrony.

Area of Assessment

Balance and gait

ICF Domain

Activity

Time to Administer

Ten minutes

Equipment

A video recording device

Reference Values

VanSwearningen et al[124] reported the mean total score and subset mean scores of those with and without a history of falls for 52 community-dwelling, frail, older male veterans (mean age 74.8 years, range = 61 to 95 years) who ambulated without assistive devices other than a straight cane (Table 5.15.1).

TABLE 5.15.1. MODIFIED GAIT ABNORMALITY RATING SCALE REFERENCE VALUES FOR COMMUNITY-DWELLING, OLDER ADULTS					
GARS-M SCORE	RECURRENT FALLS (N = 36)		NO RECURRENT FALLS (N = 16)		ALL (N = 52)	
	X	SD	X	SD	X	SD
	9.0	4.59	3.8	3.37	7.42	4.87

Minimal Detectable Change

Not established

Minimal Clinically Important Difference

Not established

Cut-Off Scores

A cut-off score of 9 differentiated between fallers and nonfallers in a group of community-dwelling, frail, elderly men with 62.3% sensitivity and 87.1% specificity.[126]

Psychometric Properties

Reliability

Intrarater reliability of 3 raters for 2 trials in community-dwelling, older, frail adults produced ICCs of 0.968, 0.950, and 0.984, while interrater reliability across 2 trials produced Kappa statistics of 0.577 and 0.603 for the total GARS-M scores.[124]

Hale et al[127] reported **good** intrarater reliability with ICC = 0.7 in 9 people with moderate to severe intellectual disability. GARS-M scores for a group of subjects with conversion disorders were quantified with good to excellent intrarater reliability (ICC = 0.989) and interrater reliability (ICC = 0.878).[128]

Concurrent Validity

Huang and colleagues[129] demonstrated the validity of the GARS-M scale in a group of elderly women with a variety of diagnoses by comparing GARS-M scores with stance time variability recorded on a computerized walkway (Gait-Mat II [E.Q., Inc]). The observational rating had sensitivity of 81% and specificity of 53%.[129]

Stride length and walking speed had **excellent** negative correlations ($r = -0.754$, $r = -0.679$, respectively) with the GARS-M in community-dwelling, elderly adults.[124] In other words, higher GARS-M scores corresponded to shorter strides and slower walking speed.[124]

Mean GARS-M scores distinguished between frail, older people with and without a history of recurrent falls (mean GARS-M scores of 9.0 and 3.8, respectively).

Responsiveness/Sensitivity to Change

Not established

5.16: References

1. Rehabilitation Measures Database. http://www.rehabmeasures.org/rehabweb/allmeasures.aspx?PageView=Shared. Published 2010. Accessed March 10, 2016.
2. Podsiadlo D, Richardson S. The timed "Up & Go": a test of basic functional mobility for frail elderly persons. *J Am Geriatr Soc.* 1991;39(2):142-148.
3. Guideline for the prevention of falls in older persons. American Geriatrics Society, British Geriatrics Society, and American Academy of Orthopaedic Surgeons Panel on Falls Prevention. *J Am Geriatr Soc.* 2001;49(5):664-672.
4. Bischoff HA, Stahelin HB, Monsch AU, et al. Identifying a cut-off point for normal mobility: a comparison of the timed 'up and go' test in community-dwelling and institutionalised elderly women. *Age Ageing.* 2003;32(3):315-320.
5. Bohannon RW. Reference values for the timed up and go test: a descriptive meta-analysis. *J Geriatr Phys Ther.* 2006;29(2):64-68.
6. Pondal M, del Ser T. Normative data and determinants for the timed "up and go" test in a population-based sample of elderly individuals without gait disturbances. *J Geriatr Phys Ther.* 2008;31(2):57-63.
7. Steffen TM, Hacker TA, Mollinger L. Age- and gender-related test performance in community-dwelling elderly people: six-minute walk test, Berg balance scale, timed up & go test, and gait speeds. *Phys Ther.* 2002;82(2):128-137.

8. Ries JD, Echternach JL, Nof L, Gagnon Blodgett M. Test-retest reliability and minimal detectable change scores for the timed "up & go" test, the six-minute walk test, and gait speed in people with Alzheimer disease. *Phys Ther.* 2009;89(6):569-579.

9. Flansbjer UB, Holmback AM, Downham D, Patten C, Lexell J. Reliability of gait performance tests in men and women with hemiparesis after stroke. *J Rehabil Med.* 2005;37(2):75-82.

10. Dal Bello-Haas V, Klassen L, Sheppard MS, Metcalfe A. Psychometric properties of activity, self-efficacy, and quality-of-life measures in individuals with Parkinson's disease. *Physiother Can.* 2011;63(1):47-57.

11. Wright AA, Cook CE, Baxter GD, Dockerty JD, Abbott JH. A comparison of 3 methodological approaches to defining major clinically important improvement of 4 performance measures in patients with hip osteoarthritis. *J Orthop Sports Phys Ther.* 2011;41(5):319-327.

12. Shumway-Cook A, Brauer S, Woollacott M. Predicting the probability for falls in community-dwelling older adults using the timed up & go test. *Phys Ther.* 2000;80(9):896-903.

13. Barry E, Galvin R, Keogh C, Horgan F, Fahey T. Is the timed up and go test a useful predictor of risk of falls in community dwelling older adults: a systematic review and meta-analysis. *BMC Geriatr.* 2014;14:14.

14. Beauchet O, Fantino B, Allali G, Muir SW, Montero-Odasso M, Annweiler C. Timed up and go test and risk of falls in older adults: a systematic review. *J Nutr Health Aging.* 2011;15(10):933-938.

15. Rydwik E, Bergland A, Forséén L, Fräändin K. Psychometric properties of timed up and go in elderly people: a systematic review. *Physical & Occupational Therapy in Geriatrics.* 2011;29(2):102-125.

16. Schoene D, Wu SM, Mikolaizak AS, et al. Discriminative ability and predictive validity of the timed up and go test in identifying older people who fall: systematic review and meta-analysis. *J Am Geriatr Soc.* 2013;61(2):202-208.

17. Andersson AG, Kamwendo K, Seiger A, Appelros P. How to identify potential fallers in a stroke unit: validity indexes of 4 test methods. *J Rehabil Med.* 2006;38(3):186-191.

18. Whitney JC, Lord SR, Close JC. Streamlining assessment and intervention in a falls clinic using the timed up and go test and physiological profile assessments. *Age Ageing.* 2005;34(6):567-571.

19. Thomas JI, Lane JV. A pilot study to explore the predictive validity of 4 measures of falls risk in frail elderly patients. *Arch Phys Med Rehabil.* 2005;86(8):1636-1640.

20. Dite W, Connor HJ, Curtis HC. Clinical identification of multiple fall risk early after unilateral transtibial amputation. *Arch Phys Med Rehabil.* 2007;88(1):109-114.

21. Nocera JR, Stegemoller EL, Malaty IA, et al. Using the timed up & go test in a clinical setting to predict falling in Parkinson's disease. *Arch Phys Med Rehabil.* 2013;94(7):1300-1305.

22. Dibble LE, Lange M. Predicting falls in individuals with Parkinson's disease: a reconsideration of clinical balance measures. *J Neurol Phys Ther.* 2006;30(2):60-67.

23. Arnold CM, Faulkner RA. The history of falls and the association of the timed up and go test to falls and near-falls in older adults with hip osteoarthritis. *BMC Geriatr.* 2007;7:17.

24. Whitney SL, Marchetti GF, Schade A, Wrisley DM. The sensitivity and specificity of the timed "up & go" and the dynamic gait index for self-reported falls in persons with vestibular disorders. *J Vestib Res.* 2004;14(5):397-409.

25. Kennedy DM, Stratford PW, Wessel J, Gollish JD, Penney D. Assessing stability and change of four performance measures: a longitudinal study evaluating outcome following total hip and knee arthroplasty. *BMC Musculoskelet Disord.* 2005;6:3.

26. Katz-Leurer M, Rotem H, Lewitus H, Keren O, Meyer S. Functional balance tests for children with traumatic brain injury: within-session reliability. *Pediatr Phys Ther.* 2008;20(3):254-258.

27. Steffen T, Seney M. Test-retest reliability and minimal detectable change on balance and ambulation tests, the 36-item short-form health survey, and the unified Parkinson's disease rating scale in people with parkinsonism. *Phys Ther.* 2008;88(6):733-746.

28. van Hedel HJ, Wirz M, Dietz V. Assessing walking ability in subjects with spinal cord injury: validity and reliability of 3 walking tests. *Arch Phys Med Rehabil.* 2005;86(2):190-196.

29. Bennie S, Bruner K, Dizon A, Fritz H, Goodman B, Peterson S. Measurement of balance: comparison of the timed "up and go" test and functional reach test with the Berg balance scale. *J Phys Ther Sci.* 2003;15(2):93-97.

30. Nordin E, Lindelof N, Rosendahl E, Jensen J, Lundin-Olsson L. Prognostic validity of the timed up-and-go test, a modified get-up-and-go test, staff's global judgement and fall history in evaluating fall risk in residential care facilities. *Age Ageing.* 2008;37(4):442-448.

31. Wrisley DM, Kumar NA. Functional gait assessment: concurrent, discriminative, and predictive validity in community-dwelling older adults. *Phys Ther.* 2010;90(5):761-773.

32. Brusse KJ, Zimdars S, Zalewski KR, Steffen TM. Testing functional performance in people with Parkinson's disease. *Phys Ther.* 2005;85(2):134-141.

33. Meretta BM, Whitney SL, Marchetti GF, Sparto PJ, Muirhead RJ. The five times sit to stand test: responsiveness to change and concurrent validity in adults undergoing vestibular rehabilitation. *J Vestib Res.* 2006;16(4-5):233-243.

34. Sabirli F, Paker N, Bugdayci D. The relationship between knee injury and osteoarthritis outcome score (KOOS) and timed up and go test in patients with symptomatic knee osteoarthritis. *Rheumatol Int.* 2013;33(10):2691-2694.

35. Lemay JF, Nadeau S. Standing balance assessment in ASIA D paraplegic and tetraplegic patients: concurrent validity of the Berg balance scale. *Spinal Cord.* 2010;48(3):245-250.

36. Lin MR, Hwang HF, Hu MH, Wu HD, Wang YW, Huang FC. Psychometric comparisons of the timed up and go, one-leg stand, functional reach, and Tinetti balance measures in community-dwelling older people. *J Am Geriatr Soc.* 2004;52(8):1343-1348.

37. French HP, Fitzpatrick M, FitzGerald O. Responsiveness of physical function outcomes following physiotherapy intervention for osteoarthritis of the knee: an outcome comparison study. *Physiotherapy.* 2011;97(4):302-308.

38. Hofheinz M, Schusterschitz C. Dual task interference in estimating the risk of falls and measuring change: a comparative, psychometric study of four measurements. *Clin Rehabil.* 2010;24(9):831-842.

39. Caixeta GC, Dona F, Gazzola JM. Cognitive processing and body balance in elderly subjects with vestibular dysfunction. *Braz J Otorhinolaryngol.* 2012;78(2):87-95.

40. Campbell CM, Rowse JL, et al. The effect of cognitive demand on timed up and go performance in older adults with and without Parkinson disease. *J Neurol Phys Ther.* 2003;27(1):2-7.

41. Maranhao-Filho PA, Maranhao ET, Lima MA, Silva MM. Rethinking the neurological examination II: dynamic balance assessment. *Arq Neuropsiquiatr.* 2011;69(6):959-963.

42. Elazzazi A, Chapman N, Murphy E, White R. Measurement of distance walked and physiologic responses to a 6-minute walk test on level ground and on a treadmill: a comparative study. *J Geriatr Phys Ther.* 2012;35(1):2-7.

43. Brooks D, Solway S, Gibbons WJ. ATS statement on six-minute walk test. *Am J Respir Crit Care Med.* 2003;167(9):1287.

44. Lusardi MM, Pellecchia GL, Schulman M. Functional performance in community living older adults. *J Geriatr Phys Ther.* 2003;26(3):14-22.

45. Cahalin LP, Mathier MA, Semigran MJ, Dec GW, DiSalvo TG. The six-minute walk test predicts peak oxygen uptake and survival in patients with advanced heart failure. *Chest.* 1996;110(2):325-332.

46. Casanova C, Cote CG, Marin JM, et al. The 6-min walking distance: long-term follow up in patients with COPD. *Eur Respir J.* 2007;29(3):535-540.

47. Wevers LE, Kwakkel G, van de Port IG. Is outdoor use of the six-minute walk test with a global positioning system in stroke patients' own neighbourhoods reproducible and valid? *J Rehabil Med.* 2011;43(11):1027-1031.

48. Perera S, Mody SH, Woodman RC, Studenski SA. Meaningful change and responsiveness in common physical performance measures in older adults. *J Am Geriatr Soc.* 2006;54(5):743-749.

49. Redelmeier DA, Bayoumi AM, Goldstein RS, Guyatt GH. Interpreting small differences in functional status: the six minute walk test in chronic lung disease patients. *Am J Respir Crit Care Med.* 1997;155(4):1278-1282.

50. Eng JJ, Dawson AS, Chu KS. Submaximal exercise in persons with stroke: test-retest reliability and concurrent validity with maximal oxygen consumption. *Arch Phys Med Rehabil.* 2004;85(1):113-118.

51. Lam T, Noonan VK, Eng JJ. A systematic review of functional ambulation outcome measures in spinal cord injury. *Spinal Cord.* 2008;46(4):246-254.

52. Rasekaba T, Lee AL, Naughton MT, Williams TJ, Holland AE. The six-minute walk test: a useful metric for the cardiopulmonary patient. *Intern Med J.* 2009;39(8):495-501.

53. Forrest GF, Hutchinson K, Lorenz DJ, et al. Are the 10 meter and 6 minute walk tests redundant in patients with spinal cord injury? *PLoS One.* 2014;9(5):e94108.

54. Kosak M, Smith T. Comparison of the 2-, 6-, and 12-minute walk tests in patients with stroke. *J Rehabil Res Dev.* 2004;41(1):103.

55. Scivoletto G, Tamburella F, Laurenza L, Foti C, Ditunno JF, Molinari M. Validity and reliability of the 10-m walk test and the 6-min walk test in spinal cord injury patients. *Spinal Cord.* 2011;49(6):736-740.

56. Tappen RM, Roach KE, Buchner D, Barry C, Edelstein J. Reliability of physical performance measures in nursing home residents with Alzheimer's disease. *J Gerontol A Biol Sci Med Sci.* 1997;52(1):M52-55.

57. Mossberg KA. Reliability of a timed walk test in persons with acquired brain injury. *Am J Phys Med Rehabil.* 2003;82(5):385-390; quiz 391-382.

58. van Loo MA, Moseley AM, Bosman JM, de Bie RA, Hassett L. Test-re-test reliability of walking speed, step length and step width measurement after traumatic brain injury: a pilot study. *Brain Inj.* 2004;18(10):1041-1048.

59. Harada ND, Chiu V, Stewart AL. Mobility-related function in older adults: assessment with a 6-minute walk test. *Arch Phys Med Rehabil.* 1999;80(7):837-841.

60. Connelly DM, Thomas BK, Cliffe SJ, Perry WM, Smith RE. Clinical utility of the 2-minute walk test for older adults living in long-term care. *Physiother Can.* 2009;61(2):78-87.

61. Gijbels D, Alders G, Van Hoof E, et al. Predicting habitual walking performance in multiple sclerosis: relevance of capacity and self-report measures. *Mult Scler.* 2010;16(5):618-626.

62. Gijbels D, Eijnde BO, Feys P. Comparison of the 2- and 6-minute walk test in multiple sclerosis. *Mult Scler.* 2011;17(10):1269-1272.

63. Hiengkaew V, Jitaree K, Chaiyawat P. Minimal detectable changes of the Berg balance scale, Fugl-Meyer assessment scale, timed "up & go" test, gait speeds, and 2-minute walk test in individuals with chronic stroke with different degrees of ankle plantarflexor tone. *Arch Phys Med Rehabil.* 2012;93(7):1201-1208.

64. Rossier P, Wade DT. Validity and reliability comparison of 4 mobility measures in patients presenting with neurologic impairment. *Arch Phys Med Rehabil.* 2001;82(1):9-13.

65. Resnik L, Borgia M. Reliability of outcome measures for people with lower-limb amputations: distinguishing true change from statistical error. *Phys Ther.* 2011;91(4):555-565.

66. Leung AS, Chan KK, Sykes K, Chan KS. Reliability, validity, and responsiveness of a 2-min walk test to assess exercise capacity of COPD patients. *Chest.* 2006;130(1):119-125.

67. Miller PA, Moreland J, et al. Measurement properties of a standardized version of the two-minute walk test for individuals with neurological dysfunction. *Physiother Can.* 2002;5(4):241-248.

68. Brooks D, Hunter JP, Parsons J, Livsey E, Quirt J, Devlin M. Reliability of the two-minute walk test in individuals with transtibial amputation. *Arch Phys Med Rehabil.* 2002;83(11):1562-1565.

69. Brooks D, Davis AM, Naglie G. Validity of 3 physical performance measures in inpatient geriatric rehabilitation. *Arch Phys Med Rehabil.* 2006;87(1):105-110.

70. Kosak M, Smith T. Comparison of the 2-, 6-, and 12-minute walk tests in patients with stroke. *J Rehabil Res Dev.* 2005;42(1):103-107.

71. Salavati M, Mazaheri M, Khosrozadeh F, Mousavi SM, Negahban H, Shojaei H. The Persian version of locomotor capabilities index: translation, reliability and validity in individuals with lower limb amputation. *Qual Life Res.* 2011;20(1):1-7.

72. Brooks D, Davis AM, Naglie G. The feasibility of six-minute and two-minute walk tests in in-patient geriatric rehabilitation. *Can J Aging.* 2007;26(2):159-162.

73. Brooks D, Parsons J, Hunter JP, Devlin M, Walker J. The 2-minute walk test as a measure of functional improvement in persons with lower limb amputation. *Arch Phys Med Rehabil.* 2001;82(10):1478-1483.

74. Gijbels D, Dalgas U, Romberg A, et al. Which walking capacity tests to use in multiple sclerosis? A multicentre study providing the basis for a core set. *Mult Scler.* 2012;18(3):364-371.

75. Brooks D, Parsons J, Tran D, et al. The two-minute walk test as a measure of functional capacity in cardiac surgery patients. *Arch Phys Med Rehabil.* 2004;85(9):1525-1530.

76. Shumway-Cook A, Baldwin M, Polissar NL, Gruber W. Predicting the probability for falls in community-dwelling older adults. *Phys Ther.* 1997;77(8):812-819.

77. Shumway-Cook A, Gruber W, Baldwin M, Liao S. The effect of multidimensional exercises on balance, mobility, and fall risk in community-dwelling older adults. *Phys Ther.* 1997;77(1):46-57.

78. Vereeck L, Wuyts F, Truijen S, Van de Heyning P. Clinical assessment of balance: normative data, and gender and age effects. *Int J Audiol.* 2008;47(2):67-75.

79. Romero S, Bishop MD, Velozo CA, Light K. Minimum detectable change of the Berg Balance Scale and Dynamic Gait Index in older persons at risk for falling. *J Geriatr Phys Ther.* 2011;34(3):131-137.

80. Cattaneo D, Jonsdottir J, Repetti S. Reliability of four scales on balance disorders in persons with multiple sclerosis. *Disabil Rehabil.* 2007;29(24):1920-1925.

81. Jonsdottir J, Cattaneo D. Reliability and validity of the dynamic gait index in persons with chronic stroke. *Arch Phys Med Rehabil.* 2007;88(11):1410-1415.

82. Lin JH, Hsu MJ, Hsu HW, Wu HC, Hsieh CL. Psychometric comparisons of 3 functional ambulation measures for patients with stroke. *Stroke.* 2010;41(9):2021-2025.

83. Huang SL, Hsieh CL, Wu RM, Tai CH, Lin CH, Lu WS. Minimal detectable change of the timed "up & go" test and the dynamic gait index in people with Parkinson disease. *Phys Ther.* 2011;91(1):114-121.

84. Hall CD, Herdman SJ. Reliability of clinical measures used to assess patients with peripheral vestibular disorders. *J Neurol Phys Ther.* 2006;30(2):74-81.

85. Pardasaney PK, Latham NK, Jette AM, et al. Sensitivity to change and responsiveness of four balance measures for community-dwelling older adults. *Phys Ther.* 2012;92(3):388-397.

86. Balasubramanian CK. The community balance and mobility scale alleviates the ceiling effects observed in the currently used gait and balance assessments for the community-dwelling older adults. *J Geriatr Phys Ther.* 2015;38(2):78-89.

87. Pardasaney PK, Ni P, Slavin MD, et al. Computer-adaptive balance testing improves discrimination between community-dwelling elderly fallers and nonfallers. *Arch Phys Med Rehabil.* 2014;95(7):1320-1327. e1321.

88. Landers MR, Backlund A, Davenport J, Fortune J, Schuerman S, Altenburger P. Postural instability in idiopathic Parkinson's disease: discriminating fallers from nonfallers based on standardized clinical measures. *J Neurol Phys Ther.* 2008;32(2):56-61.

89. Cattaneo D, Regola A, Meotti M. Validity of six balance disorders scales in persons with multiple sclerosis. *Disabil Rehabil.* 2006;28(12):789-795.

90. Whitney SL, Hudak MT, Marchetti GF. The dynamic gait index relates to self-reported fall history in individuals with vestibular dysfunction. *J Vestib Res.* 2000;10(2):99-105.

91. Jonsson LR, Kristensen MT, Tibaek S, Andersen CW, Juhl C. Intra- and interrater reliability and agreement of the Danish version of the Dynamic Gait Index in older people with balance impairments. *Arch Phys Med Rehabil.* 2011;92(10):1630-1635.

92. McConvey J, Bennett SE. Reliability of the Dynamic Gait Index in individuals with multiple sclerosis. *Arch Phys Med Rehabil.* 2005;86(1):130-133.

93. Wrisley DM, Walker ML, Echternach JL, Strasnick B. Reliability of the dynamic gait index in people with vestibular disorders. *Arch Phys Med Rehabil.* 2003;84(10):1528-1533.

94. Cakit BD, Saracoglu M, Genc H, Erdem HR, Inan L. The effects of incremental speed-dependent treadmill training on postural instability and fear of falling in Parkinson's disease. *Clin Rehabil.* 2007;21(8):698-705.

95. Marchetti GF, Whitney SL. Construction and validation of the 4-item dynamic gait index. *Phys Ther.* 2006;86(12):1651-1660.

96. Morgan MT, Friscia LA, Whitney SL, Furman JM, Sparto PJ. Reliability and validity of the Falls Efficacy Scale-International (FES-I) in individuals with dizziness and imbalance. *Otol Neurotol.* 2013;34(6):1104-1108.

97. Shumway-Cook A, Taylor CS, Matsuda PN, Studer MT, Whetten BK. Expanding the scoring system for the Dynamic Gait Index. *Phys Ther.* 2013;93(11):1493-1506.

98. Matsuda PN, Taylor CS, Shumway-Cook A. Evidence for the validity of the modified dynamic gait index across diagnostic groups. *Phys Ther.* 2014;94(7):996-1004.

99. Walker ML, Austin AG, Banke GM, et al. Reference group data for the functional gait assessment. *Phys Ther.* 2007;87(11):1468-1477.

100. Marchetti GF, Lin CC, Alghadir A, Whitney SL. Responsiveness and minimal detectable change of the dynamic gait index and functional gait index in persons with balance and vestibular disorders. *J Neurol Phys Ther.* 2014;38(2):119-124.

101. Leddy AL, Crowner BE, Earhart GM. Functional gait assessment and balance evaluation system test: reliability, validity, sensitivity, and specificity for identifying individuals with Parkinson disease who fall. *Phys Ther.* 2011;91(1):102-113.

102. Thieme H, Ritschel C, Zange C. Reliability and validity of the functional gait assessment (German version) in subacute stroke patients. *Arch Phys Med Rehabil.* 2009;90(9):1565-1570.

103. Ellis T, Cavanaugh JT, Earhart GM, Ford MP, Foreman KB, Dibble LE. Which measures of physical function and motor impairment best predict quality of life in Parkinson's disease? *Parkinsonism Relat Disord.* 2011;17(9):693-697.

104. Gill TM, Williams CS, Tinetti ME. Assessing risk for the onset of functional dependence among older adults: the role of physical performance. *J Am Geriatr Soc.* 1995;43(6):603-609.

105. Dai B, Ware WB, Giuliani CA. A structural equation model relating physical function, pain, impaired mobility (IM), and falls in older adults. *Arch Gerontol Geriatr.* 2012;55(3):645-652.

106. Schenkman M, Cutson TM, Kuchibhatla M, Chandler J, Pieper C. Reliability of impairment and physical performance measures for persons with Parkinson's disease. *Phys Ther.* 1997;77(1):19-27.

107. Franzen E, Paquette C, Gurfinkel VS, Cordo PJ, Nutt JG, Horak FB. Reduced performance in balance, walking and turning tasks is associated with increased neck tone in Parkinson's disease. *Exp Neurol.* 2009;219(2):430-438.

108. Schenkman M, Ellis T, Christiansen C, et al. Profile of functional limitations and task performance among people with early- and middle-stage Parkinson disease. *Phys Ther.* 2011;91(9):1339-1354.

109. Shiu CH, Ng SS, Kwong PW, Liu TW, Tam EW, Fong SS. Timed 360 degrees Turn Test for Assessing People With Chronic Stroke. *Arch Phys Med Rehabil.* 2016;97(4):536-544.

110. Tager IB, Swanson A, Satariano WA. Reliability of physical performance and self-reported functional measures in an older population. *J Gerontol A Biol Sci Med Sci.* 1998;53(4):M295-300.

111. Berg K. Measuring balance in the elderly: preliminary development of an instrument. *Physiother Can.* 1989;41(6):304-311.

112. Shubert TE, Schrodt LA, Mercer VS, Busby-Whitehead J, Giuliani CA. Are scores on balance screening tests associated with mobility in older adults? *J Geriatr Phys Ther.* 2006;29(1):35-39.

113. Dite W, Temple VA. Development of a clinical measure of turning for older adults. *Am J Phys Med Rehabil.* 2002;81(11):857-866; quiz 867-858.

114. Gill TM, Williams CS, Mendes de Leon CF, Tinetti ME. The role of change in physical performance in determining risk for dependence in activities of daily living among nondisabled community-living elderly persons. *J Clin Epidemiol.* 1997;50(7):765-772.

115. Dite W, Temple VA. A clinical test of stepping and change of direction to identify multiple falling older adults. *Arch Phys Med Rehabil.* 2002;83(11):1566-1571.

116. Blennerhassett JM, Jayalath VM. The Four Square Step Test is a feasible and valid clinical test of dynamic standing balance for use in ambulant people poststroke. *Arch Phys Med Rehabil.* 2008;89(11):2156-2161.

117. Duncan RP, Earhart GM. Four square step test performance in people with Parkinson disease. *J Neurol Phys Ther.* 2013;37(1):2-8.

118. Whitney SL, Marchetti GF, Morris LO, Sparto PJ. The reliability and validity of the Four Square Step Test for people with balance deficits secondary to a vestibular disorder. *Arch Phys Med Rehabil.* 2007;88(1):99-104.

119. Holden MK, Gill KM, Magliozzi MR. Gait assessment for neurologically impaired patients. Standards for outcome assessment. *Phys Ther.* 1986;66(10):1530-1539.

120. Sanchez-Blanco I, Ochoa-Sangrador C, Lopez-Munain L, Izquierdo-Sanchez M, Fermoso-Garcia J. Predictive model of functional independence in stroke patients admitted to a rehabilitation programme. *Clin Rehabil.* 1999;13(6):464-475.

121. Kollen B, Kwakkel G, Lindeman E. Time dependency of walking classification in stroke. *Phys Ther.* 2006;86(5):618-625.

122. Mehrholz J, Wagner K, Rutte K, Meissner D, Pohl M. Predictive validity and responsiveness of the functional ambulation category in hemiparetic patients after stroke. *Arch Phys Med Rehabil.* 2007;88(10):1314-1319.

123. Holden MK, Gill KM, Magliozzi MR, Nathan J, Piehl-Baker L. Clinical gait assessment in the neurologically impaired. Reliability and meaningfulness. *Phys Ther.* 1984;64(1):35-40.

124. VanSwearingen JM, Paschal KA, Bonino P, Yang JF. The modified Gait Abnormality Rating Scale for recognizing the risk of recurrent falls in community-dwelling elderly adults. *Phys Ther.* 1996;76(9):994-1002.

125. Wolfson L, Whipple R, Amerman P, Tobin JN. Gait assessment in the elderly: a gait abnormality rating scale and its relation to falls. *J Gerontol.* 1990;45(1):M12-M19.

126. VanSwearingen JM, Paschal KA, Bonino P, Chen TW. Assessing recurrent fall risk of community-dwelling, frail older veterans using specific tests of mobility and the physical performance test of function. *J Gerontol A Biol Sci Med Sci.* 1998;53(6):M457-M464.

127. Hale L, McIlraith L, Miller C, Stanley-Clarke T, George R. The interrater reliability of the modified gait abnormality rating scale for use with people with intellectual disability. *J Intellect Dev Disabil.* 2010;35(2):77-81.

128. Vandenberg JM, George DR, O'Leary AJ, Olson LC, Strassburg KR, Hollman JH. The modified gait abnormality rating scale in patients with a conversion disorder: a reliability and responsiveness study. *Gait Posture.* 2015;41(1):125-129.

129. Huang WN, VanSwearingen JM, Brach JS. Gait variability in older adults: observational rating validated by comparison with a computerized walkway gold standard. *Phys Ther.* 2008;88(10):1146-1153.

Chapter 6

Pathological Gait

6.1: INTRODUCTION TO OBSERVATIONAL GAIT ANALYSIS

Observational gait analysis (OGA) is a critical skill that requires practice to accurately identify deviations and develop hypotheses of each deviation's probable cause. Under the mentorship of Dr. Jacquelin Perry, the Pathokinesiology Service and Physical Therapy Department at Rancho Los Amigos National Rehabilitation Center (Downey, California) developed the Full Body Gait Analysis Form, composed of 178 check-off options for identifying both major and minor deviations during an observational analysis.[1] In an effort to simplify the form, while maintaining the ability to identify important major deviations, the authors of this manual developed a new, abbreviated form (JAKC OGA form with 66 check off options). The form also includes measurement of walking speed (the sixth vital sign),[2,3] stride length, and cadence with normative gender and age comparisons (% normal).[4] Once gait deviations are documented, a problem solving approach is initiated to determine probable cause of each deviation and differentiate primary and secondary deficits from useful compensatory substitutions. The clinician develops hypotheses regarding probable causes of deviations, and then plans and performs the examination based on these hypotheses. Examination results are then evaluated with input from the patient/client and family to identify impairments, activity limitations, and participation restrictions (International Classification of Functioning, Disability and Health [ICF]).[5] Together with the client and family, the clinician then sets realistic treatment goals and intervention plans.

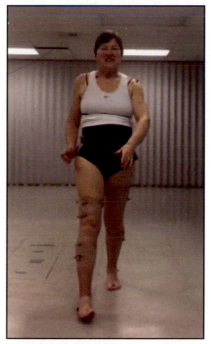

Figure 6-1. Frontal plane observational gait analysis

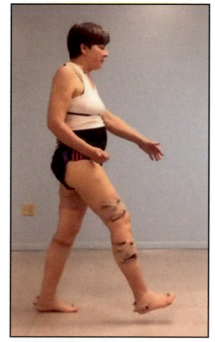

Figure 6-2. Sagittal plane observational gait analysis

Adams JM, Cerny K.
Observational Gait Analysis: A Visual Guide (pp 143-170).
© 2018 SLACK Incorporated.

6.2: Overview: Observational Analysis Process

a. Observe the patient/client's gait from both sagittal and frontal views. You may choose to videotape the individual making sure the recording device is oriented at 90 degrees to the subject in both sagittal and frontal planes (see section 6.3).

b. Identify the major deviations (using the JAKC OGA form) and document assistive devices used.

c. Determine temporal and spatial parameters (10-Meter Walk Test [10MWT]) as baseline measures for treatment outcomes.

   i. Velocity (value and % normal)

   ii. Cadence (value and % normal)

   iii. Stride length (value and % normal)

d. Develop hypotheses of the likely causes (impairments) of the observed deviations (see section 6.4).

e. Based on hypotheses, plan and perform a clinical examination to determine impairments, activity limitations, and participation restrictions.

f. Evaluate the examination results and determine the cause of the deviations (impairments, secondary deviations, or compensatory strategies).

g. Together with the family and patient/client, set reasonable goals, develop and implement a treatment plan including the use of adaptive, assistive, orthotic, prosthetic, protective, or supportive equipment.

h. Re-examine the patient/client and evaluate the effectiveness of the therapeutic intervention.

6.3: Procedures for Determining Major Gait Deviations

a. Either directly observe or obtain consent to videotape the patient/client.

   i. If possible the patient/client should walk barefoot to allow analysis without the influence of a shoe or orthotic.

   ii. If possible minimal, tight clothing should be worn to view as much of the body and limbs as they feel comfortable exposing. Suggested clothing would include, sports bra, bicycle shorts, bathing suit, or gym attire.

b. Instruct the client to walk at a comfortable speed (self-selected) and, if possible, a fast but safe speed.

c. Observe the client's walking from multiple views (anterior, posterior, right, and left sides). Videotape if possible.

d. Identify prominent gait deviations that interfere with activity and participation restrictions.

e. Determine the reference limb for analysis (most involved).

f. Identify the deviations on the JAKC OGA form.

   i. Start at the foot and proceed proximally.

g. Identify the deviations within the context of the essential accomplishments of weight acceptance, single limb support, and swing limb advancement.

6.4: Causes of Observed Gait Deviations

Causes may be:

a. **Primary:** Deviations directly caused by an impairment

  i. The ICF Classification System defines an impairment as the "loss or abnormality of physiological, psychological or anatomical structure or function at the organ system level."[5]

  ii. Most impairments that affect gait can be fit into 4 major categories for observational analysis.[6]

    1. Deformity

    2. Weakness

    3. Impaired motor control

    4. Pain

  iii. Examples

    1. Excess dorsiflexion (DF) in Mid Stance due to weak calf muscles

    2. Contralateral pelvic drop due to weak hip abductors

b. **Secondary:** Deviations that result from an abnormal posture at an adjacent joint

  i. Examples

    1. Excess DF in Mid Stance due to a knee flexion contracture rather than weak calf muscles. The knee flexion contracture is the primary deviation.

    2. Forefoot contact at Initial Contact due to inadequate knee extension in Terminal Swing, rather than a plantar flexion (PF) contracture. Lack of full knee extension is the cause of this deviation.

c. **Compensatory:** Deviations that are useful postural movements that accommodate for an impairment, rather than being a direct result of an impairment

  i. Examples

    1. Excess hip flexion in Mid Swing to compensate for weak dorsiflexors to assure toe clearance.

    2. Ipsilateral trunk lean in stance to compensate for weak hip abductors.

6.5: Impairments in Persons With Musculoskeletal Disorders

- Pain
- Skeletal deformity
- Muscle weakness (strength or power production)
- Range of motion (muscle/joint stiffness, contractures, hypomobility)
- Joint laxity
- Sensory deficits (light touch, proprioception)
- Impaired motor control
  - Movement speed
  - Timing

- ○ Coordination
- ○ Balance and postural control
- Impaired cardiac function (endurance)
- Impaired circulatory function
- Impaired respiratory function
- Impaired hormonal and nutritional factors
- Impaired psychosocial factors

Diagnostic Groups

- Injuries that may include:
  - ○ Sprains, strains, tendonosis, fractures, dislocations, overuse, peripheral nerve injury
- Degenerative diseases (osteoarthritis)
- Systemic diseases (rheumatoid arthritis)
- History of poliomyelitis
- Spina bifida
- Guillain-Barre syndrome
- Muscular dystrophy

6.6: IMPAIRMENTS IN PERSONS WITH CENTRAL NERVOUS SYSTEM DISORDERS

Primary Impairments

a. Motor system impairments
  - Muscle weakness
  - State of the motor neuron pool
    - ○ Hypertonicity
      - ◆ Spasticity
      - ◆ Rigidity
      - ◆ Hyper-reflexia
    - ○ Hypotonicity
  - Coordination impairments
    - ○ Activation and sequencing impairments
      - ◆ Abnormal synergies
      - ◆ Coactivation
      - ◆ Impaired interjoint coordination

- Timing impairments
  - ◆ Movement initiation and termination
  - ◆ Scaling forces (dysmetria)
  - ◆ Involuntary movements
- Dystonia
- Associated movements
- Tremor
- Choreiform and athetoid movements

b. Sensory system impairments
- Somatosensory deficits
  - Discriminative touch
  - Proprioception
  - Pain
  - Temperature
- Visual deficits
- Vestibular deficits

c. Cognitive and perceptual impairments
- Body image impairments
- Spatial relationship impairments
- Apraxia
- Attention
- Orientation
- Memory
- Problem solving
- Level of consciousness

Diagnostic Groups

- Stroke
- Multiple sclerosis
- Spinal cord injury
- Traumatic or acquired brain injury
- Parkinson's disease
- Cerebral palsy
- Amyotrophic lateral sclerosis

6.7: MAJOR DEVIATIONS AND IMPAIRMENTS: ANKLE, FOOT, AND TOES

JAKC OGA Form

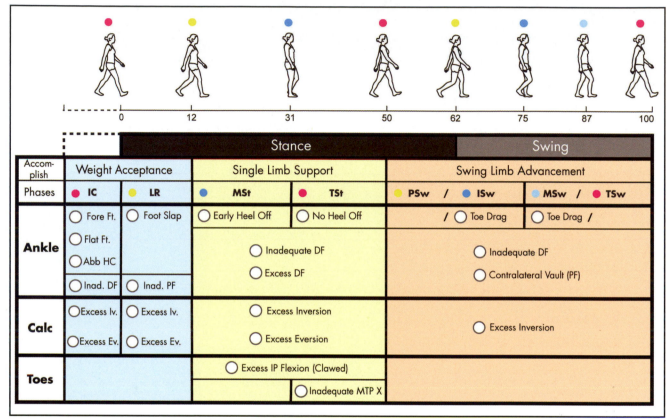

Figure 6-3. JAKC OGA form: ankle, foot, and toe deviations.

Major Deviations in Each Essential Accomplishment

Weight Acceptance:

Single Limb Support:

Swing Limb Advancement:

TABLE 6-1. GAIT DEVIATION DEFINITIONS (ANKLE, FOOT, AND TOES)	
DEVIATION "DATED TERMINOLOGY"	**DEFINITION**
Forefoot Contact (Fore Ft)	Initial ground contact made with the forefoot
Flatfoot Contact (Flat Ft)	Initial ground contact made with both the hindfoot and forefoot
Abbreviated Heel Contact (Abb HC)	At Initial Contact, the interval of heel only is shortened
Foot Slap	Rapid PF after heel strike; often audible as forefoot hits ground
Inadequate Dorsiflexion	Less than normal DF for the phase
Excess Dorsiflexion	More than normal DF for the phase
Inadequate Plantar Flexion	Less than normal PF for the phase
Excess Inversion (Iv) "Pes Cavus"	More than normal calcaneal or forefoot inversion for the phase(s)
Excess Eversion (Ev) "Pes Planus"	More than normal calcaneal or forefoot eversion for the phase(s)
Early Heel Off	Heel off in Mid Stance
No Heel Off	Heel does not rise in Terminal Stance
Inadequate Metatarsophalangeal (MTP) Extension (Inadequate MTP X)	Less than normal MTP extension in Terminal Stance and Pre-Swing
Excess Interphalangeal (IP) Flexion "Clawed"	More than normal IP Flexion of toes with MTP extension (hammer toes) or without (clawed toes) MTP extension
Toe Drag	Contact of foot with the ground during Initial or Mid Swing
Contralateral Vault (PF)	Excess ankle PF with prolonged forefoot weight bearing of the contralateral stance limb during reference limb swing limb advancement

TABLE 6-2. ANKLE, FOOT, AND TOE DEVIATIONS WITH POSSIBLE IMPAIRMENTS

DEVIATIONS: ANKLE	GAIT PHASE	POSSIBLE CAUSES
Abbreviated Heel Contact (Abb HC) Video: CS 001 R Side WB **Flatfoot Contact (Flat Ft)** Video: CS 004 Post CU	Initial Contact	**Primary** • Weak dorsiflexors (MMT < 3/5) • PF contracture/hypomobility • Impaired motor control (abnormal plantar flexor activity) **Secondary** • To inadequate knee extension in Terminal Swing • To a knee flexion contracture • Impaired motor control (abnormal hamstring activity) **Compensatory** • To reduce or avoid the effects of the heel rocker due to weak quadriceps (decreasing the knee flexion moment)
Forefoot Contact (Fore Ft) Video: CS 005_Barefoot_L Side WB	Initial Contact	**Primary** • See Inadequate Dorsiflexion • See Inadequate Knee Extension • Combination of both Inadequate Dorsiflexion and Inadequate Knee Extension **Compensatory** • To accommodate for a shorter limb • To avoid heel pain
Foot Slap Video: CS 006 R Side WB	Loading Response	**Primary** • Weak dorsiflexors (MMT 3/5) when heel contact at Initial Contact occurs
Excess Dorsiflexion	Mid and Terminal Stance	**Primary** • Weak plantar flexors **Secondary** • To excess hip and/or knee flexion **Compensatory** • To lower contralateral limb for Initial Contact

(continued)

TABLE 6-2 (CONTINUED). ANKLE, FOOT, AND TOE DEVIATIONS WITH POSSIBLE IMPAIRMENTS

DEVIATIONS: ANKLE	GAIT PHASE	POSSIBLE CAUSES
Inadequate Dorsiflexion Video: CS 004 L Side WB	Initial Contact	**Primary** • Weak dorsiflexors (MMT < 3/5) • Impaired motor control (abnormal plantar flexor activity) • PF contracture/hypomobility • Ankle pain, joint effusion
	Mid and Terminal Stance	**Primary** • PF contracture (rigid) • Impaired motor control (plantar flexor spasticity and/or extensor synergy) • Ankle pain, joint effusion, ankle fusion **Compensatory** • To avoid the ankle rocker secondary to weak plantar flexors reducing an external DF moment
Video: CS 005_Barefoot_L Side WB	Swing	**Primary** • Weak dorsiflexors (MMT < 3/5) • PF contracture/hypomobility • Impaired motor control (abnormal plantar flexor activity)
Inadequate Plantar Flexion	Loading	**Secondary** • To an abbreviated or absent heel rocker
Early Heel Off	Mid Stance	**Primary** • Skeletal deformity • Impaired motor control (over activity of plantar flexors) • PF contracture/hypomobility **Secondary** • To excess knee flexion **Compensatory** • Voluntary PF to accommodate for a short reference limb

(continued)

TABLE 6-2 (CONTINUED). ANKLE, FOOT, AND TOE DEVIATIONS WITH POSSIBLE IMPAIRMENTS		
DEVIATIONS: ANKLE	**GAIT PHASE**	**POSSIBLE CAUSES**
No Heel Off Video: CS 002 R Side WB	**Terminal Stance**	**Primary** • Weak plantar flexors (MMT < 4/5) • Forefoot pain **Secondary** • To inadequate toe extension • To excess ankle DF • To knee hyperextension (lack of tibial advancement)
Excess Inversion (Iv) Video: 1_A_ankle Iv-Ev angle	**Stance and Swing**	**Primary** • Skeletal deformity (hindfoot varus deformity; uncompensated forefoot varus) • Impaired motor control AT/PT or soleus activity • Equinovarus contracture/hypomobility **Secondary** • To genu varum • To hip rotational deformities
Video: CS 004 Post CU	**Swing only**	**Primary** • All of the above • Flaccid paralysis of the pretibials (AT, EHL, and EDL)
Excess Eversion (Ev)	**Stance**	**Primary** • Skeletal deformity (hindfoot valgus deformity; uncompensated forefoot valgus) • Weak invertors in loading: (anterior and posterior tibialis) **Secondary** • To a compensated forefoot varus • To a genu valgus • To hip rotational deformities **Compensatory** • For limited ankle DF range of motion to preserve forward progression (center of pressure progresses onto the medial aspect of the foot, flattening the ML arch) *(continued)*

TABLE 6-2 (CONTINUED). ANKLE, FOOT, AND TOE DEVIATIONS WITH POSSIBLE IMPAIRMENTS		
DEVIATIONS: ANKLE	**GAIT PHASE**	**POSSIBLE CAUSES**
Toe Drag Video: CS 005_Barefoot_L Side WB	Initial Swing	**Primary** • See Inadequate Knee Flexion • Impaired motor control decreasing knee flexion (abnormal rectus femoris/knee extensor activity) **Secondary** • To excess contralateral knee flexion
	Mid Swing	**Primary** • Inadequate DF; weak dorsiflexors (MMT < 3/5) **Secondary** • To inadequate hip flexion (see Table 6-8) • To excess contralateral knee flexion
Contralateral Vault (PF)	Swing	**Compensatory** Voluntary contralateral PF (heel rise or toe walking) to lengthen stance limb and achieve swing limb toe clearance when there is: • A longer swing limb • Inadequate knee flexion in Initial Swing • Inadequate DF in Mid Swing
MTP/TOES		
Excess IP Flexion "Clawed"	Stance	**Primary** • Skeletal deformity • Toe contractures • Impaired motor control (abnormal FDL and FHL muscle activity) • Weak intrinsic muscles **Compensatory** • For a weak soleus and gastrocnemius to increase plantar flexor force to control tibial advancement
Inadequate MTP Extension (Inadequate MTP X)	Terminal Stance and Pre-Swing	**Primary** • Skeletal Deformity: Hallux Rigidus • Impaired motor control (abnormal FHL and FDL muscle activity) **Secondary** • To avoid forefoot pain (avoiding forefoot and toe rockers) • To no heel off

MMT: Manual Muscle test; AT: anterior tibialis; PT: posterior tibialis; EHL: extensor hallucis longus; EDL: extensor digitorum longus; ML: medial longitudinal; FDL: flexor digitorum longus; FHL: flexor hallucis longus

6.8: Major Deviations and Impairments: Knee

JAKC OGA Form

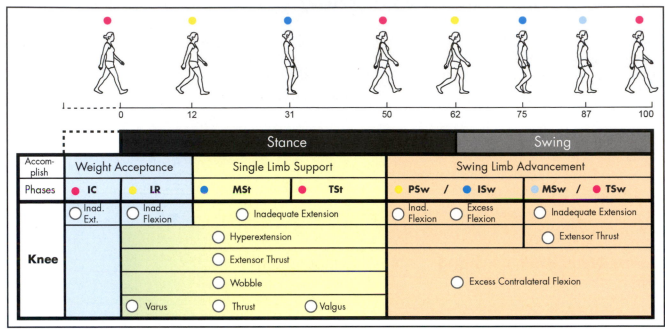

Figure 6-4. JAKC OGA form: knee deviations.

Major Deviations in Each Essential Accomplishment

Weight Acceptance:

Single Limb Support:

Swing Limb Advancement:

TABLE 6-3. GAIT DEVIATION DEFINITIONS (KNEE)	
DEVIATION **"DATED TERMINOLOGY"**	**DEFINITION**
Inadequate Extension **(Excess Flexion)** **In Stance: "Crouch Gait"**	Less than normal extension for the phase
Inadequate Flexion **In Swing: "Stiff-Legged Gait"**	Less than normal flexion for the phase
Hyperextension **"Back Knee"**	Extension beyond neutral
Extensor Thrust	Rapid movement toward extension
Wobble	Repeated alternating flexion and extension
Varus **"Bow-Leg"**	Adduction of distal tibia relative to femur
Valgus **"Knock-Knee"**	Abduction of distal tibia relative to femur
Varus/Valgus Thrust	Rapid movement into varus or valgus
Excess Contralateral Flexion	Contralateral flexion during reference swing limb advancement

TABLE 6-4. KNEE DEVIATIONS WITH POSSIBLE IMPAIRMENTS

DEVIATIONS: KNEE	GAIT PHASE	POSSIBLE CAUSES
Inadequate Extension Video: 2_knee Fl-Ext angle	Stance	**Primary** • Knee flexion contracture/hypomobility • Impaired motor control (abnormal knee flexor activity) • Knee pain • Joint effusion **Secondary** • To excess DF posture • To excess hip flexion posture
Video: 2_knee Fl-Ext angle	Swing	**Primary** • Weak quadriceps • Knee flexion contracture/hypomobility • Impaired motor control (abnormal knee flexor activity) • Knee pain • Joint effusion **Compensatory** • To allow for forefoot or flatfoot contact *(continued)*

TABLE 6-4 (CONTINUED). KNEE DEVIATIONS WITH POSSIBLE IMPAIRMENTS

DEVIATIONS: KNEE	GAIT PHASE	POSSIBLE CAUSES
Inadequate Flexion Video: CS 004 R Side WB	Loading	**Primary** • Weak quadriceps • Impaired motor control (abnormal quadriceps activity) • Impaired proprioception • Tibiofemoral and/or patellofemoral pain • Skeletal deformity **Secondary** • To a PF posture • To abnormal plantar flexor muscle activity • To a forefoot or flatfoot contact **Compensatory** • For anterior cruciate ligament deficiency
	Swing	**Primary** • Impaired motor control (abnormal RF/knee extensor activity) • Tibiofemoral and/or patellofemoral pain • Skeletal deformity **Secondary** • To inadequate hip flexion • To inadequate knee flexion in Pre-Swing • To inadequate hip extension in Terminal Stance • To "no heel off" in Terminal Stance
Excess Flexion Video: CS 004 L Side WB	Swing	**Primary** • Impaired motor control (abnormal hip and knee flexor activity) **Compensatory** • To assure toe clearance

(continued)

Table 6-4 (continued). Knee Deviations With Possible Impairments

DEVIATIONS: KNEE	GAIT PHASE	POSSIBLE CAUSES
Hyperextension Video: CS 004 R Side WB	Stance	**Primary** • Weak quadriceps • Impaired motor control (abnormal knee extensor) • Impaired proprioception **Secondary** • To a PF posture **Compensatory** • To increase limb stability with weak quadriceps and plantar flexors
Extensor Thrust	Stance	**Primary** • Weak quadriceps • Impaired motor control (abnormal knee extensor; abnormal plantar flexor activity) • Impaired proprioception **Secondary** • To a PF contracture with forefoot contact at Initial Contact **Compensatory** • To increase limb stability with weak quadriceps
Video: CS 001 R Side WB	Swing	**Compensatory** • To assure knee extension in Terminal Swing in preparation for Initial Contact (when quadriceps are weak)
Wobble Video: 5BF_knee Fl-Ext angle	Stance	**Primary** • Impaired proprioception • Impaired motor control (abnormal knee extensor activity; abnormal plantar flexor activity) *(continued)*

TABLE 6-4 (CONTINUED). KNEE DEVIATIONS WITH POSSIBLE IMPAIRMENTS

DEVIATIONS: KNEE	GAIT PHASE	POSSIBLE CAUSES
Varus Video: 3_P_knee Var-Val angle	Stance	**Primary** • Skeletal deformity • Ligamentous laxity/joint instability • Degenerative joint changes (osteoarthritis) **Secondary** • To an uncompensated hindfoot varus deformity • To a compensated forefoot valgus deformity
Valgus	Stance	**Primary** • Skeletal deformity • Ligamentous laxity/joint instability • Degenerative joint changes (rheumatoid arthritis) **Secondary** • To an uncompensated hindfoot valgus deformity • To a compensated forefoot varus deformity • To an ipsilateral trunk lean
Varus/Valgus Thrust Video: 3_P_knee Var-Val mom	Stance	**Primary** • Skeletal deformity • Ligamentous/joint instability
Excess Contralateral Flexion Video: CS 002 R Side WB	Swing	**Primary** • Any factor that causes stance limb knee flexion on the contralateral limb **Secondary** • To intentionally lower the shorter reference swing limb to the ground for Initial Contact

RF: rectus femoris

6.9: Major Deviations and Impairments: Thigh

JAKC OGA Form

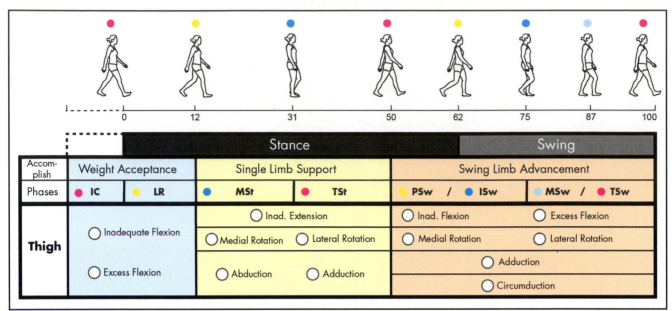

Figure 6-5. JAKC OGA form: thigh deviations.

Major Deviations in Each Essential Accomplishment

Weight Acceptance:

Single Limb Support:

Swing Limb Advancement:

TABLE 6-5. GAIT DEVIATION DEFINITIONS (THIGH)	
DEVIATION **"DATED TERMINOLOGY"**	**DEFINITION**
Inadequate Extension **"Crouched Gait"**	Inadequate extension in Stance Phase
Inadequate Flexion	Less than normal flexion for the phase
Excess Flexion **"Steppage Gait"**	More than normal flexion for Swing Phase
Medial Rotation	Position of the femur with femoral condyles facing medially
Lateral Rotation	Position of the femur with femoral condyles facing laterally
Abduction	Abduction of the femur beyond neutral
Adduction **"Scissoring Gait"**	Adduction of the femur beyond neutral
Circumduction	Thigh abduction with flexion followed by adduction during swing limb advancement

TABLE 6-6. THIGH DEVIATIONS WITH POSSIBLE IMPAIRMENTS

DEVIATIONS: THIGH	GAIT PHASE	POSSIBLE CAUSES
Inadequate Extension Video: 2_thigh Fl-Ext angle	Stance	**Primary** • Hip flexion contracture/hypomobility • Joint arthrodesis • Impaired motor control (abnormal hip flexor muscle activity) • Hip pain • Hip joint effusion **Secondary** • To excess knee flexion, excess DF posture • To "no heel off" in Terminal Stance
Inadequate Flexion Video: 5BF_thigh Fl-Ext angle	Initial Contact and Loading Response	**Primary** • Impaired motor control • Skeletal deformity **Secondary** • To inadequate hip flexion in Terminal Swing **Compensatory** • To decrease demand on weak hip extensors in Loading Response
	Swing	**Primary** • Weak hip flexors • Impaired motor control (weak flexion synergy; abnormal hamstring activity) **Secondary** • To toe drag **Compensatory** • To decrease demand on hip extensors in preparation for Initial Contact and Loading
Excess Flexion Video: 6_thigh Fl-Ext angle	Swing	**Compensatory** • For inadequate knee flexion in Initial Swing for toe clearance • For inadequate DF in Mid Swing for toe clearance • For a longer swing limb • For CL knee flexion, which functionally shortens the stance limb

(continued)

TABLE 6-6 (CONTINUED). THIGH DEVIATIONS WITH POSSIBLE IMPAIRMENTS		
DEVIATIONS: THIGH	**GAIT PHASE**	**POSSIBLE CAUSES**
Medial Rotation Video: 1_A_thigh MR-LR angle	Stance and Swing	**Primary** • Skeletal deformity: femoral anteversion • Impaired motor control (abnormal medial rotator muscle activity; adductor longus and brevis, medial hamstrings) • Medial rotation contracture/hypomobility **Compensatory** • In stance, to increase knee stability when the quadriceps are weak
Lateral Rotation Video: 5BF_P_thigh MR-LR angle	Stance	**Primary** • Skeletal deformity: femoral retroversion • Lateral rotation contracture/hypomobility **Compensatory** • To progress center of mass forward when DF range of motion is inadequate
	Swing	**Compensatory** • For toe clearance when DF is inadequate • To advance limb using hip adductors when hip flexors are weak
Abduction	Stance	**Primary** • Skeletal deformity **Secondary** • To a pelvic obliquity • To a contralateral pelvic hike • To a spinal deformity (scoliosis) • To increase base of support for stability • To advance limb when hip flexors are weak (circumduct) **Compensatory** • For longer reference limb (LL discrepancy)
	Swing	**Compensatory** • To clear a longer swing limb (true LL discrepancy) • To clear a functionally longer swing limb (inadequate hip or knee flexion, inadequate DF)

(continued)

TABLE 6-6 (CONTINUED). THIGH DEVIATIONS WITH POSSIBLE IMPAIRMENTS		
DEVIATIONS: THIGH	**GAIT PHASE**	**POSSIBLE CAUSES**
Adduction	Stance and Swing	**Primary** • Skeletal deformity • Adduction contracture/hypomobility • Impaired motor control (abnormal adductor muscle activity) **Secondary** • To pelvic obliquity • To a CL pelvic drop • To a spinal deformity
Circumduction Video: CS 001 Ant WB	Swing	**Compensatory** • To advance limb and clear foot when hip flexion, knee flexion, and/or DF are inadequate
CL: contralateral; LL: leg length		

6.10: MAJOR DEVIATIONS AND IMPAIRMENTS: PELVIS AND TRUNK

Major Deviations in Each Essential Accomplishment

Weight Acceptance:

Single Limb Support:

Swing Limb Advancement:

JAKC OGA Form

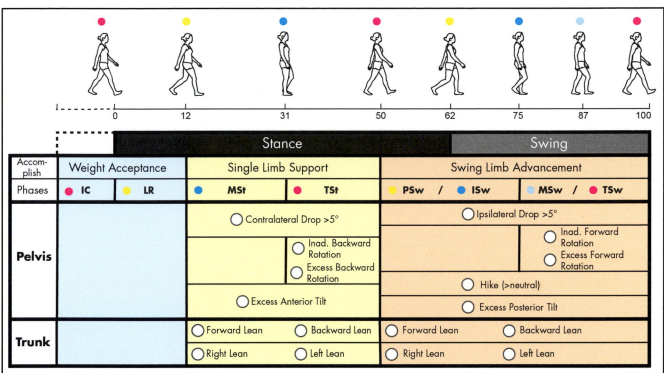

Figure 6-6. JAKC OGA form: pelvis and trunk deviations.

TABLE 6-7. GAIT DEVIATION DEFINITIONS (PELVIS)	
DEVIATION **"DATED TERMINOLOGY"**	**DEFINITION**
Contralateral Drop ***"Trendelenburg Gait"***	>5 degrees drop of iliac crest on swing limb during stance on the reference limb
Ipsilateral Drop	>5 degrees drop of iliac crest on reference swing limb during stance on the contralateral limb
Hike	Elevation of iliac crest of reference limb above neutral during swing limb advancement
Excess Backward Rotation ***"Retracted Pelvis"***	>5 degrees backward rotation during Terminal Stance, which may continue into Pre- and Initial Swing
Inadequate Backward Rotation	Less backward rotation (<5 degrees) during Terminal Stance
Inadequate Forward Rotation	Less forward rotation (<5 degrees) during Mid and Terminal Swing
Excess Forward Rotation	>5 degrees forward rotation during Mid and Terminal Swing
Excess Anterior Tilt	More than normal anterior tilt of pelvis
Excess Posterior Tilt	Any posterior tilt of pelvis from the normal posture of anterior tilt

TABLE 6-8. PELVIC DEVIATIONS WITH POSSIBLE IMPAIRMENTS

DEVIATIONS: PELVIS	GAIT PHASE	POSSIBLE CAUSES
Contralateral Drop (> 5 degrees) Video: 2_A_pelv R-L drop angle	Stance	**Primary** • Weak hip abductors on reference limb • Impaired motor control (abnormal adductor muscle activity) of reference limb • Adduction contracture on reference limb **Secondary** • To a skeletal deformity • To a pelvic obliquity **Compensatory** • For a short CL leg (LL discrepancy)
Ipsilateral Drop (> 5 degrees)	Swing	**Primary** • Weak contralateral hip abductors • Impaired motor control (abnormal CL adductor muscle activity) • CL adduction contracture **Secondary** • To a skeletal deformity • To a pelvic obliquity **Compensatory** • For a short reference limb (LL discrepancy)
Hike Video: 5BF_P_pelv R-L drop angle	Swing	**Compensatory** • For toe clearance when there is inadequate knee flexion in Pre- and Initial Swing or inadequate hip flexion and DF in Mid Swing
Inadequate Forward Rotation Video: 2_T_pelv F-B rot angle	Swing	**Primary** • Impaired motor control (abnormal activity of trunk, pelvis, and hip muscles) **Secondary** • To inadequate contralateral backward rotation **Compensatory** • To decrease demand on weak hip extensors and knee extensors during Loading Response
Excess Forward Rotation Video: 7_pelv F-B rot angle	Swing	**Secondary** • To excess contralateral backward rotation **Compensatory** • To advance limb when hip flexors are weak *(continued)*

DEVIATIONS: PELVIS	GAIT PHASE	POSSIBLE CAUSES
Excess Backward Rotation Video: 2_T_pelv F-B rot angle	Terminal Stance	**Primary** • Impaired motor control (inability to perform selective activation of trunk, pelvis, hip, and/or plantar flexor muscles) **Secondary** • To contralateral excess forward rotation **Compensatory** • To progress over a plantar flexed foot • To achieve a trailing limb with limited thigh extension in Terminal Stance (hip flexion contracture) • To achieve a trailing limb when there is no heel off in Terminal Stance (weak plantar flexors)
Inadequate Backward Rotation	Terminal Stance	**Primary** • Impaired motor control (inability to perform selective activation of trunk, pelvis, hip, and/or plantar flexor muscles) **Secondary** • To contralateral inadequate forward rotation • To inadequate thigh extension
Excess Anterior Tilt Video: 7_pelv A-P tilt angle	Stance	**Primary** • Hip flexion contracture/hypomobility • Impaired motor control (abnormal hip flexor muscle activity) • Weak hip extensor and/or abdominal muscles **Secondary** • To a forward trunk lean
Excess Posterior Tilt Video: 2_pelv A-P tilt angle	Stance	**Primary** • Hamstring tightness/contracture • Impaired motor control (abnormal hamstring muscle activity) **Secondary** • To a backward trunk lean
	Swing	**Secondary** • To advance the limb when hip flexors are weak

TABLE 6-8 (CONTINUED). PELVIC DEVIATIONS WITH POSSIBLE IMPAIRMENTS

LL: leg length

JAKC OGA Form

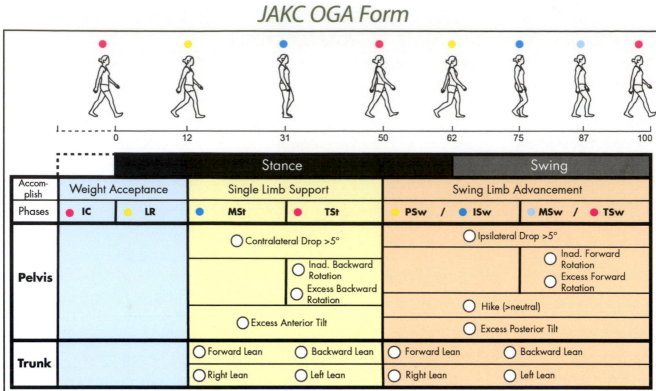

Figure 6-6. JAKC OGA form: pelvis and trunk deviations.

TABLE 6-9. GAIT DEVIATION DEFINITIONS (TRUNK)	
DEVIATION **"DATED TERMINOLOGY"**	**DEFINITION**
Forward Lean	Anterior lean of the trunk past vertical
Backward Lean **"Gluteus Maximus Gait"**	Posterior lean of the trunk past vertical
Right Lean **"Gluteus Medius Gait"** **Bilateral: "Waddling Gait"**	Right lean of the trunk past vertical
Left Lean **"Gluteus Medius Gait"** **Bilateral: "Waddling Gait"**	Left lean of the trunk past vertical

TABLE 6-10. TRUNK DEVIATIONS WITH POSSIBLE IMPAIRMENTS

DEVIATIONS: TRUNK	GAIT PHASE	POSSIBLE CAUSES
Forward Lean Video: 6_trunk F-B lean angle	Stance	**Primary** • Skeletal deformity • Impaired postural control (inadequate hip and spine extensor muscle activity) **Secondary** • To a pelvic anterior tilt posture • To using an assistive device • To excess hip flexion **Compensatory** • To progress over a plantar flexed foot • To move GRFV anterior to knee when knee extensors are weak to improve limb stability • To improve visual input when sensation is impaired
Backward Lean Video: 7_trunk F-B lean angle	Stance	**Compensatory** • To increase hip extension moment reducing demand for weak hip extensors
	Swing	**Primary** • To advance limb when hip flexors are weak
Right Lean Video: 1_P_trunk R-L lean angle	Stance	**Primary** • Skeletal deformity (scoliosis, pelvic obliquity) • Impaired postural control **Secondary** • To using an assistive device with right UE **Compensatory** • To reduce hip adduction moment decreasing demand on weak right hip abductor muscles • To decrease right hip pain • To clear left swing limb when there is inadequate hip and/or knee flexion or inadequate DF • To clear left swing limb with LL discrepancy (long left limb) • To reduce CL (left) pelvic drop

(continued)

TABLE 6-10 (CONTINUED). TRUNK DEVIATIONS WITH POSSIBLE IMPAIRMENTS		
DEVIATIONS: TRUNK	GAIT PHASE	POSSIBLE CAUSES
Left Lean Video: 5BF_trunk R-L lean angle Video: 2_P_trunk R-L lean angle	Stance	**Primary** • Skeletal deformity (scoliosis, pelvic obliquity) • Impaired postural control **Secondary** • To using an assistive device with left UE **Compensatory** • To reduce hip adduction moment decreasing demand on weak left hip abductor muscles • To decrease left hip pain • To clear right swing limb when there is inadequate hip and/or knee flexion or inadequate DF • To clear right swing limb with LL discrepancy (long right limb) • To reduce CL (right) pelvic drop
GRFV: ground reaction force vector; UE: upper extremity		

6.11: REFERENCES

1. Pathokinesiology Laboratory and Department of Physical Therapy. *Observational Gait Analysis*. 4th ed. Rancho Los Amigos National Rehabilitation Center, Downey, CA: Los Amigos Research and Educational Institute Inc; 2001.
2. Fritz S, Lusardi M. White paper: "walking speed: the sixth vital sign." *J Geriatr Phys Ther.* 2009;32(2):46-49.
3. Middleton A, Fritz SL, Lusardi M. Walking speed: the functional vital sign. *J Aging Phys Act.* 2015;23(2):314-322.
4. Waters RL, Lunsford BR, Perry J, Byrd R. Energy-speed relationship of walking: standard tables. *J Orthop Res.* 1988;6(2):215-222.
5. World Health Organization. *World Health Organization International Classification of Functioning, Disability and Health: ICF.* Geneva. 2001.
6. Perry J, Burnfield JM. *Gait Analysis: Normal & Pathological Gait.* 2nd ed. Thorofare, NJ: SLACK Incorporated; 2010.

Please see videos on the accompanying website at

www.healio.com/books/oga

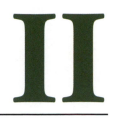

Case Studies

Instructions for Case Studies

1. Students should review the History and Evaluation for each case study.

2. Students should review the Main Videos for each case study. These are located on the book's companion website, and there are multiple views for each case study.

3. Students should access the JAKC OGA Form, located in Appendix A and on the book's companion website. Students should: fill out this form to the best of their ability; summarize deviations under "Essential Accomplishments;" and calculate velocity, cadence, and stride length under "Stride Characteristics" (based on the 10MWT outcomes in the History and Evaluation Results), comparing results to age- and gender-matched normal persons in the Appendices B and C.

4. After completing the JAKC OGA form, students should review the related Polygon Videos (skeleton, graphs, and videos) for each case study. These are also located on the book's companion website, and there are multiple views for each case study.

5. Using Chapter 6 of the text, students should consider possible causes of each deviation identified and determine which are probable causes, considering diagnosis, history, and evaluation results. Students should then generate a gait analysis report within the text, which should reflect problem solving by identifying gait deviations with probable cause.

6. Students may generate goals based on the diagnosis and evaluation results. Although goals are not included in the OGA process, this is a subsequent step leading to intervention and would be a desirable task for students to undertake.

7. Students may also consider recommending functional tests to include in the evaluation process using Chapter 5 of the text.

8. *(For Instructors)* To determine the accuracy of students' gait assessments, instructors should:

   a. Access the JAKC OGA Forms filled out by 3 expert gait analysis examiners, located on efaculty lounge, and compare students' results to expert examiners' results.

   b. Access the Final Reports generated by the expert examiners, also located on efaculty lounge.

   c. If desired, access the Gait Analysis Report Rubric in Appendix D for grading students' reports.

Adams JM, Cerny K.
Observational Gait Analysis: A Visual Guide (p 173).
© 2018 SLACK Incorporated.

Case Study 001

History and Evaluation

Patient/Client's Name: CS 001   **Gender:** Female   **DOB:** 01/12/1949   **Age:** 67

Gait Evaluation Date: 3/14/2016

Medical Diagnosis: Left stroke with R hemiparesis

Onset Date: 9/10/2010

Guide to PT Practice Pattern:

5D: Impaired motor function and sensory integrity associated with nonprogressive disorders of the CNS acquired in adolescence or adulthood.

History:

Client 001 is a 67-year-old woman who experienced a left stroke on 9/10/2010 resulting in right-sided hemiparesis and expressive aphasia. She currently walks independently without an assistive device or orthoses. She lives in a 2-story home with her husband, with 7 stairs between floors. She states that she is independent in most activities of daily living (ADL), is able to ascend and descend stairs with use of handrails, and able to enter and exit her home independently. She is right-hand dominant and has limited RUE ROM and strength with minimal volitional movement. Client 001 requires assistance with bilateral hand activities such as zippers, lacing shoes, and donning her hand splint. She enjoys traveling and being active outside with her husband; they are both retired. She is no longer a fall risk (TUG-R 10.83 sec), but has a history of falls in the past. Prior to the stroke, she was independent in ambulation and all ADL, and was very active enjoying paddle boarding 3.5 miles 4x/week, yoga 6x/week, biking, and swimming. Her goals include improving her walking speed and right UE function so that she can return to the activities she enjoyed before her stroke. She is currently participating in speech therapy and physical therapy in California State University, Long Beach's pro-bono clinics (Long Beach, California). To date, the client believes she has made "tremendous progress" since her stroke 6 years ago and is highly motivated to continue her therapy.

Past Medical History:

Two myocardial infarctions (1995 and 07/20/1998), CABG with mammary graft (08/06/1998), GERD (diagnosed 09/2001), vitreous detachment (11/23/08), atrial fibrillation (diagnosed 01/2005), severe migraines, and cataracts (removed in 2013).

Adams JM, Cerny K.
Observational Gait Analysis: A Visual Guide (pp 175-179).
© 2018 SLACK Incorporated.

Summary of Gait Deviations

Reference Limb: Right LE

Condition: Barefoot

Essential Accomplishments

Weight Acceptance (Initial Contact and Loading Response):

Single Limb Support (Mid Stance and Terminal Stance):

Swing Limb Advancement (Pre-Swing, Initial Swing, Mid Swing, and Terminal Swing):

Upper Extremity (Reciprocal Arm Swing):

Foot/Floor Contact Pattern (Barefoot):

Evaluation Results

ICF Domain: Activity

1. 10-Meter Walk Test (10MWT)

> Results: traversed 6 m in 8.6 seconds and took 12 steps

STRIDE CHARACTERISTICS: BAREFOOT AT SELF-SELECTED SPEED		
Gait speed		% N*
Cadence		% N*
Stride length (R)		% N*
*Waters; normal values for senior women 60 to 80 years		

Perry's Functional Walking Category:

ICF Domain: Body Function (Impairment Measures)

1. Upright Motor Control Test (UMCT)

MOTION	RIGHT LE (SYNERGY)
Cadence	
Hip flexion	2 (Moderate)
Knee flexion	1 (Weak)
Ankle dorsiflexion	1 (Weak)
UMCT Extension	
Hip extension	2 (Moderate)
Knee extension	1 (Weak)
Plantar flexion	2 (Moderate)
Key: 1 = Weak, 2 = Moderate, 3 = Strong	

2. Fugl-Meyer Lower Extremity Assessment (FMA-LE)

MOTION	RIGHT LE (SYNERGY)
Supine: Flexion Synergy	
Hip flexion	2 (Full motion)
Knee flexion	2 (Full motion)
Ankle dorsiflexion	2 (Full motion
Sidelying: Extension Synergy	
Hip extension	2 (Full motion)
Hip adduction	2 (Full motion)
Knee extension	2 (Full motion)
Plantar flexion	2 (Full motion)
Sitting: Movement Combining Synergies	
Knee flexion	2 (Beyond 90 degrees)
Dorsiflexion	1 (Incomplete active motion)
Standing: Movement Out of Synergy	
Knee flexion	1 (Less than 90 degrees)
Ankle dorsiflexion	1 (Partial motion)

Results: Fugl-Meyer Assessment-Lower Extremity Score 19/22

- Demonstrates full motion in synergy (supine and sidelying)
- Partial movement combining synergies (sitting)
- Partial movement out of synergy (standing)

3. Spasticity (Modified Ashworth Scale)

Hamstrings	1+
Rectus femoris	0
Knee extensors	0
Plantar flexors with knee extended	2
Invertors	0

R Striatal Hallux: excess dorsiflexion of the hallux

No proprioceptive loss at knee or ankle

4. Passive Range of Motion (PROM):

R Hip and R Knee: WNL

R Ankle:

Supine DF with knee extension: -12 degrees

Supine DF with knee flexion: 0 to 4 degrees

Weightbearing DF: 0 to 12 degrees

ICF Domain: Activity

1. Timed Up and Go (TUG-R) 10.83 seconds (no longer a fall risk)
2. mDGI: 49/64
3. Wolf Motor Function Test (WMFT): 39/85
4. Fugl-Meyer (UE): 31/66

ICF Domain: Participation

1. Stroke Impact Scale (SIS)

- Strength: 68.75%
- Memory and thinking: 92.8%
- Emotion: 100%
- Communication 90%
- ADL/IADL: 77.5%
- Mobility: 97.2%
- Hand function: 30%
- Participation role function: 100%
- Overall stroke recovery: 80%

Additional Recommendations
1. Mini-Mental State Examination (MMSE): 27/30

Examiner:

Print Name: Janet M. Adams, PT   Date: 4/12/2016   License: CA PT 11023

Signature: *Janet M. Adams, PT*

Examiner:

Print Name: Kay Cerny, PT   Date: 4/12/2016   License: CA PT 558

Signature: *Kay Cerny, PT*

Please see videos on the accompanying website at

www.healio.com/books/oga

Case Study 002

History and Evaluation

Patient/Client's Name: CS 002   **Gender:** Female   **DOB:** 07/11/1960   **Age:** 55

Gait Evaluation Date: 3/28/2016

Medical Diagnosis: Benign brain tumor excision with R hemiparesis 1 week later

Onset Date: 2/16/2010

Guide to PT Practice Pattern:

5D: Impaired motor function and sensory integrity associated with nonprogressive disorders of the CNS acquired in adolescence or adulthood.

History:

Client 002 is a 55-year-old woman who experienced a brain hemorrhage 2/16/2010 following excision of a benign brain tumor 1 week prior. She is hemiparetic on the right side and walks independently without an assistive device or orthoses. She lives alone in a one-story home with her 3 dogs, and reports that she is independent in "most activities" of daily living (ADL). She is right-hand dominant with limited RUE strength, ROM, and minimal volitional movement. She enjoys gardening and cooking and performs these activities with her left hand. She is a least-limited community ambulator and expressed a fear of being "pushed over" in a crowded environment. She states she currently has no difficulty with fall recovery and reported her last fall was in 2010. Prior to the brain hemorrhage, Client 002 was a software engineer, independent with all ADL, and was extremely active traveling, hiking, and cycling with friends. Her goals include improving her walking speed and right UE function for activities such as washing her hair and unscrewing a jar lid. She is currently participating at California State University, Long Beach's pro-bono neuro clinic (Long Beach, California) and is highly motivated to continue her physical therapy.

Past Medical History:

Benign brain tumor excised 2/09/2010 with brain hemorrhage 1 week later.

Adams JM, Cerny K.
Observational Gait Analysis: A Visual Guide (pp 181-185).
© 2018 SLACK Incorporated.

SUMMARY OF GAIT DEVIATIONS

Reference Limb: Right LE

Condition: Barefoot

Essential Accomplishments

Weight Acceptance (Initial Contact and Loading Response):

Single Limb Support (Mid Stance and Terminal Stance):

Swing Limb Advancement (Pre-Swing, Initial Swing, Mid Swing, and Terminal Swing):

Upper Extremity (Reciprocal Arm Swing):

Foot/Floor Contact Pattern (Barefoot):

EVALUATION RESULTS

ICF Domain: Activity

1. 10-Meter Walk Test (10MWT)

    Results: traversed 4 m in 8 sec taking 12 steps

STRIDE CHARACTERISTICS: BAREFOOT AT SELF-SELECTED SPEED		
Gait speed		% N*
Cadence		% N*
Stride length (R)		% N*
*Waters; normal values for women 20 to 59 years		

    Perry's Functional Walking Category:

ICF Domain: Body Function (Impairment Measures)

1. Upright Motor Control Test (UMCT)

MOTION	RIGHT LE (SYNERGY)
UMCT Flexion	
Hip flexion	3 (Strong)
Knee flexion	2 (Moderate)
Ankle dorsiflexion	1 (Weak)
UMCT Extension	
Hip extension	2 (Moderate)
Knee extension	3 (Strong)
Plantar flexion	2 (Moderate)
Key: 1＝Weak, 2＝Moderate, 3＝Strong	

2. Fugl-Meyer Lower Extremity Assessment (FMA-LE)

MOTION	RIGHT LE (SYNERGY)
Supine: Flexion Synergy	
Hip flexion	2 (Full motion)
Knee flexion	1 (Partial motion)
Ankle dorsiflexion	2 (Full motion)
Sidelying: Extension Synergy	
Hip extension	2 (Full motion)
Hip adduction	2 (Full motion)
Knee extension	2 (Full motion)
Plantar flexion	2 (Full motion)
Sitting: Movement Combining Synergies	
Knee flexion	2 (Beyond 90 degrees)
Ankle dorsiflexion	2 (Normal)
Standing: Movement Out of Synergy	
Knee flexion	1 (Less than 90 degrees)
Ankle dorsiflexion	1 (Partial motion)

Results: Fugl-Meyer Lower Extremity Score 19/22

- Demonstrates full motion in synergy (supine and sidelying)
- Demonstrates full motion combining synergies (sitting)
- Demonstrates partial movement out of synergy (standing)

3. Muscle Strength (Manual Muscle Test [MMT])

MUSCLE GROUP	RIGHT LE
Hip extensors	3/5
Hip abductors	2+/5
Knee extensors	5/5
Plantar flexors	2+/5
Hip flexors	2+/5
Knee flexors	2+/5
Dorsiflexors	4+/5

4. Range of Motion (Muscle/Joint Stiffness) Contractures

- **No LE contractures**

5. Spasticity: (Modified Ashworth Scale)

Right elbow flexors	1+
Right wrist flexors	1+
Right plantar flexors	1
Right knee extensors	1+

6. Sensory Testing

- **No proprioceptive loss at the knee or ankle**

ICF Domain: Activity

1. Mini-BESTest: Total: 23/28

Anticipatory	4/6 (unable to stand on right leg)
Reactive postural control	6/6
Dynamic gait	7/10 (deficits in changing speed, pivot turns, obstacles)

2. Wolf Motor Function Test (WMFT): 39/85

ICF Domain: Participation

1. Stroke Impact Scale (SIS)

- Strength: 81%
- Memory and thinking: 100%
- Emotion: 67%
- Communication: 100%
- ADL/IADL: 78%
- Mobility: 89%

2. Activities-Specific Balance Confidence Scale (ABC): 79%

Examiner:

Print Name: Janet M. Adams, PT   Date: 4/12/2016   License: CA PT 11023

Signature: *Janet M. Adams, PT*

Examiner:

Print Name: Kay Cerny, PT   Date: 4/12/2016   License: CA PT 558

Signature: *Kay Cerny, PT*

Please see videos on the accompanying website at

www.healio.com/books/oga

Case Study 003

History and Evaluation

Patient/Client's Name: CS 003   **Gender:** Male   **DOB:** 03/26/1951   **Age:** 65

Gait Evaluation Date: 3/28/2016

Medical Diagnosis: Osteoarthritis (OA), R total knee replacement (TKR) in July 2012 and L TKR planned April 21, 2016 (in 1 month)

Onset Date: OA 1990s

Guide to PT Practice Pattern:

4H: Impaired joint mobility, motor function, muscle performance, and ROM associated with joint arthroplasty

4I: Bony surgery

History:

Client 003 is a 65-year-old man who underwent a right TKR in July 2012 with a planned left TKR for April 21, 2016. He walks independently without an assistive device or orthoses. He is currently employed full-time as a marine biologist and has a consulting business; both jobs involve sitting for long periods of time at a microscope with an occasional requirement to collect samples while on a boat at sea (6x/year). He lives in a one-story home with his significant other, is independent in most activities of daily living (ADL; KOOS-ADL 86.7%) and enjoys traveling, gardening, hiking, golfing, and bird watching. Although his KOOS Rec/Sports score is low (20%), he exercises 2 to 3x/week at a fitness club and reports walking on the treadmill at varying speeds and inclines for 30 minutes/trial with reports of pain at higher inclines and faster speeds. At rest he states there is no pain. He ascends/descends stairs foot over foot with 2/10 pain (VAS) on ascent and 4/10 on descent. He also has pain when walking downhill and when golfing 18 holes. His goal is to be able to travel, hike, cycle, and play golf without pain. He is in good health and highly motivated.

Past Medical History:

Right TKR July 2012 with excellent results according to client. Following the right TKR there is a leg length discrepancy of 2.2 cm (R > L). No history of hypertension, diabetes, sleep apnea, or seizure activity.

Adams JM, Cerny K.
Observational Gait Analysis: A Visual Guide (pp 187-190).
© 2018 SLACK Incorporated.

SUMMARY OF GAIT DEVIATIONS

Reference limb: Left LE

Condition: Barefoot

Essential Accomplishments

Weight Acceptance (Initial Contact and Loading Response):

Single Limb Support (Mid Stance and Terminal Stance):

Swing Limb Advancement (Pre-Swing, Initial Swing, Mid Swing, and Terminal Swing):

Upper Extremities (Reciprocal Arm Swing):

Foot/Floor Contact Pattern (Barefoot): Normal Pattern

EVALUATION RESULTS

ICF Domain: Activity

1. 10-Meter Walk Test (10MWT)

Self-Selected Gait Speed: Barefoot, L LE reference limb

Results: traversed 4 m in 3.15 sec taking 6 steps

STRIDE CHARACTERISTICS: BAREFOOT AT SELF-SELECTED SPEED		
Gait speed		% N*
Cadence		% N*
Stride length (R)		% N*
*Waters; normal values for senior men 60 to 80 years		

Perry's Functional Walking Category:

ICF Domain: Body Function (Impairment Measures)

1. Muscle Strength (Manual Muscle Test [MMT])

MUSCLE GROUP	LEFT	RIGHT
Hip F/E/Abd/Add	5/5	5/5
Quadriceps	4/5	5/5
Hamstrings	4/5	4/5
Dorsiflexors	5/5	5/5
Plantar flexors	4/5	5/5

2. Passive Range of Motion (PROM)

L knee flexion 0 to 120 degrees with pain at the extremes with approximately 5 degrees of varus alignment

3. Active Range of Motion (AROM)

L Knee flexion 0 to 100 degrees

4. Additional Impairment Measures

- Slight knee joint effusion
- Sensory deficits: none
- L Varus skeletal deformity when weightbearing (standing posture: varus 5 degrees)
- True LL discrepancy: right LE 2.2 cm longer than left LE after R TKR 07/2012
- L Varus Stress Test + (lateral collateral ligamentous laxity)
- + Anterior drawer (laxity in ACL)
- + Posterior drawer (laxity in PCL)
- + Step down with moderate pain (VAS 4/10)
- + Anterior lunge with severe pain (VAS 9/10
- + Bilateral squat: unable to do a full squat because of severe pain and ROM limitations

ICF Domain: Body Function and Activity Measure

1. Knee Injury and Osteoarthritis Outcome Score (KOOS):

- Symptoms: 57.25%
- Pain: 69.5%
- ADL: 86.7%
- Sports/Rec: 20%
- QOL: 37.5%

ICF Domain: Body Function, Activity, and Participation Measures

1. Oxford Knee Score: 39/60

> Interpretation: borderline moderate to severe osteoarthritis

2. Radiology Report:

> Prior to L TKR: 03/2016

> Radiographs: bilateral standing AP left knee reveals advanced degenerative arthritis with bone on bone spurring and sclerosis in all 3 compartments. Poor joint integrity and decreased joint space due to loss of cartilage and osteophyte formation.

> March 2016: Post R TKR and Pre L TKR

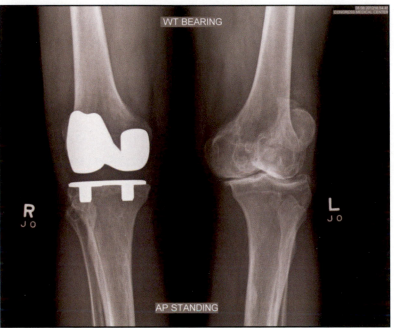

Case Figure 3-1. Anterior X-ray.

Examiner:

Print Name: Janet M. Adams, PT   Date: 4/12/2016   License: CA PT 11023

Signature: *Janet M. Adams, PT*

Examiner:

Print Name: Kay Cerny, PT   Date: 4/12/2016   License: CA PT 558

Signature: *Kay Cerny, PT*

Please see videos on the accompanying website at

www.healio.com/books/oga

Case Study 004

History and Evaluation

Patient/Client's Name: CS 004   **Gender:** Male   **DOB:** 4/3/1991   **Age:** 25

Gait Evaluation Date: 4/12/2016   **Ht:** 1.71 m   **Wt:** 229 lb

Medical Diagnosis: Rhabdomyolysis in November 2013 with bilateral anterior compartment syndrome and bilateral fasciotomies in December 2013

Onset Date: November 2013 following an intensive workout which included running several miles

Guide to PT Practice Pattern:

4I: Impaired joint mobility, motor function, muscle performance, and range of motion associated with bony or soft tissue surgery

History

Client 004 is a 25-year-old male college student who underwent bilateral anterior compartment fasciotomies in December 2013, 23 days after being diagnosed with rhabdomyolysis following an intense workout. He walks independently without an assistive device or orthoses. He states that he is not limited in any activity of daily living and currently runs, drives, and enjoys all the activities he previously experienced before the injury. He has no residual cardiopulmonary, neuromuscular, or integumentary conditions associated with the diagnosis. He will be graduating with a BS in Kinesiology from California State University, Northridge (Northridge, California) in Fall 2016.

Past Medical History

In November 2013, the client experienced bilateral "burning sensation and swelling" of both lower limbs following an intense workout, which included running where he describes himself as "pushing himself to the limit." After several hours of intense pain and swelling he went to the ER where he was admitted and diagnosed with rhabdomyolysis. While in the hospital for 23 days he developed anterior compartment syndrome, and in December 2013, underwent a bilateral anterior fasciotomy.

Medical Diagnosis Definition

Rhabdomyolysis is a syndrome caused by injury to skeletal muscle and involves leakage of large quantities of potentially toxic intracellular contents into plasma. Its final common pathway may be a disturbance in myocyte calcium homeostasis. Myoglobin is an important myocyte compound released into plasma. After muscle injury, massive plasma myoglobin levels exceed protein binding (of haptoglobin) and can precipitate in glomerular filtrate. Excess myoglobin may thus cause renal tubular obstruction, direct nephrotoxicity (ischemia and tubular injury), intrarenal vasoconstriction, and acute kidney injury (AKI).[1]

Adams JM, Cerny K.
Observational Gait Analysis: A Visual Guide (pp 191-195).
© 2018 SLACK Incorporated.

SUMMARY OF GAIT DEVIATIONS: SYMMETRICAL DEVIATIONS

Reference Limb: Right LE

Condition: Barefoot

Essential Accomplishments

Weight Acceptance (Initial Contact and Loading Response):

Single Limb Support (Mid Stance and Terminal Stance):

Swing Limb Advancement (Pre-Swing, Initial Swing, Mid Swing, and Terminal Swing):

Foot/Floor Contact Pattern (Barefoot): Normal Pattern

Upper Extremity: Normal reciprocal arm swing

Comparison of Self-Selected With Fast Walking Speed:

EVALUATION RESULTS

ICF Domain: Activity

1. 10-Meter Walk Test (10MWT)

   Results: Traversed 4 m in 4.15 sec taking 7 steps

MANUAL CALCULATIONS: SELF-SELECTED SPEED		
Gait speed		% N*
Cadence		% N*
Stride length (R)		% N*
*Waters; normal values for adult men 20 to 59 years		

   Perry's Functional Walking Category:

GAITRITE*: SELF-SELECTED SPEED

PARAMETERS	RIGHT	LEFT
Gait speed (m/sec) (m/min)	0.888 m/sec 53.28 m/min	
Cadence (steps/min)	102 steps/min	
Stride length (m)	1.05 m	1.04 m
Cycle time (sec)	1.19	1.18
Swing % GC	39.2%	41.8%
Stance % GC	60.8%	58.2%
Double limb support DLS % GC	19.2%	19.3%
Single limb support SLS % GC	41.6%	39.4%
Step/extremity ratio	0.64	0.59
Toe in (-) Toe out (+)	-1	-3

*GaitRite is manufactured by CIR Systems, Inc.

GAITRITE: FAST SPEED

PARAMETERS	RIGHT	LEFT
Velocity (m/sec) (m/min)	1.22 m/sec 73.2 m/min	
Cadence (steps/min)	114 steps/min	
Stride length (m)	1.28 m	1.30 m
Cycle time (sec)	1.05	1.06
Swing % GC	39.7%	41.0%
Stance % GC	60.4%	59.1%
Double limb support DLS % GC	19.8%	19.6%
Single limb support SLS % GC	41.4%	39.4%
Step/extremity ratio	0.76	0.76
Toe in (-) Toe out (+)	-2	-5

ICF Domain: Body Function (Impairment Measures)

1. Passive Range of Motion (PROM)

	RIGHT	LEFT
Dorsiflexion with knee extended	-18	-20
Dorsiflexion with knee flexed	-5	-5
Plantar flexion	36	35
Knee and hip	WNL	WNL

2. Muscle Strength (Manual Muscle Test [MMT])

	RIGHT	LEFT
Anterior tibialis	0/5	0/5
Extensor hallucis longus	4/5	4/5
Extensor digitorum longus	3-/5	3-/5
Soleus and gastrocnemius	18 heel rises 4/5	19 heel rises 4/5
Fibularis longus	4/5	4/5
Fibularis brevis	4/5	4/5
Quadriceps	5/5	5/5
Hamstrings	5/5	5/5
Hip (F/E, MR/LR Abd/Add)	5/5	5/5

3. Sensory Testing

Client reports occasional tingling sensation on the dorsum of the foot near the web space between toes 1 and 2 (distribution of the deep peroneal nerve). All other areas were unaffected and he was able to accurately identify light touch in the distribution of the superficial and deep peroneal nerve, common peroneal nerve, medial sural nerve, sural nerve, and tibial nerve.

4. Additional Measures: Girth and Skin Integrity

The client has significant atrophy of the anterior compartment with hypertrophy of the calf bilaterally. There are large 7-inch scars over the lateral/anterior aspect of each lower leg. The skin is a normal color, and circulation is normal.

Additional Recommendations

1. Nerve condition velocity testing, electroneuromyography to determine innervation/ denervation status of the anterior tibialis

2. Orthoses evaluation

ICF Domain: Activity

     1. 6-Minute Walk Test (6MWT)

     2. Functional Gait Assessment (FGA)

     3. Lower Extremity Functional Scale (LEFS)

ICF Domain: Participation

     1. 36-item short form survey (SF-36)

Examiner:

Print Name: Janet M. Adams, PT   Date: 4/12/2016   License: CA PT 11023

Signature: *Janet M. Adams, PT*

Examiner:

Print Name: Kay Cerny, PT   Date: 4/12/2016   License: CA PT 558

Signature: *Kay Cerny, PT*

REFERENCE

1. Muscal E. Rhabdomyolysis. *Medscape.* http://emedicine.medscape.com/article/1007814-overview. Published November 4, 2016. Accessed June 21, 2017

Please see videos on the accompanying website at

www.healio.com/books/oga

Case Study 005

History and Evaluation

Patient/Client's Name: CS 005   **Gender:** Female   **DOB:** 07/23/1997   **Age:** 18

Gait Evaluation Date: 4/22/2016

Medical Diagnosis: Transverse myelitis, inflammatory polyneuropathy

Onset Date: 4/20/2014

Guide to PT Practice Pattern:

5H: Impaired motor function, peripheral nerve integrity and sensory integrity associated with nonprogressive disorders of the spinal cord

History:

Client 005 is an 18-year-old female, college freshman who was diagnosed with transverse myelitis on April 20, 2014. She reports that initially she had significant weakness, atrophy, sensory deficits, and endurance limitations (left side more involved than right). In 2 years, she reports, there is much improvement, and she is now independent in her home environment, on campus, and in the community. She uses a light weight manual wheelchair for mobility, performs transfers, and achieves sit to stand independently. She walks short distances (50 to 100 ft) with an SPC held in her right hand using a 2-point gait pattern. She customarily wears a prefabricated "Toe-Off" ankle-foot orthosis (AFO) on the left lower extremity (LE) to assist in foot clearance during swing. She currently lives in a first-floor dorm room with a roommate. There is significant weakness in her trunk, bilateral upper extremity (UE) and LE with the left side weaker than the right. She has difficulty manipulating objects with her left hand, lacking intrinsic strength with significant atrophy present. She enjoys attending California State University's Physical Therapy Faculty Practice (Long Beach, California) 3x/week for the past 9 months and is highly motivated to exercise. Client 005 is a fall risk (TUG ~ 26 sec), but states she has not fallen in over 1 year. Prior to her diagnosis in 2014, she was "very active" enjoying hiking, dancing, and engaging in normal teenage activities. Her goals include improving walking endurance, strength, and left UE function. Her college major is Spanish, and she expressed a desire to learn several additional languages in the hopes to become an interpreter after graduation.

Past Medical History:

Unremarkable

Adams JM, Cerny K.
Observational Gait Analysis: A Visual Guide (pp 197-200).
© 2018 SLACK Incorporated.

SUMMARY OF GAIT DEVIATIONS

Condition 1: Barefoot, left LE with SPC held in right hand

Condition 2: AFO, left LE with SPC held in right hand

Essential Accomplishments:

Weight Acceptance (Initial Contact and Loading Response):

Barefoot

With Ankle-Foot Orthosis

Single Limb Support (Mid Stance and Terminal Stance):

Barefoot

With Ankle-Foot Orthosis

Swing Limb Advancement (Pre-Swing, Initial Swing, Mid Swing, and Terminal Swing):

Barefoot

With Ankle-Foot Orthosis

Upper Extremity (Reciprocal Arm Swing):

Foot/Floor Contact Pattern:

Barefoot

With Ankle-Foot Orthosis

EVALUATION RESULTS

ICF Domain: Activity

1. 10-Meter Walk Test (10MWT)

Results: Barefoot traversed 4 m in 17 sec taking 14 steps

STRIDE CHARACTERISTICS: BAREFOOT AT SELF-SELECTED SPEED		
Gait speed		% N*
Cadence		% N*
Stride length (R)		% N*
*Waters; normal values for adult women		

Perry's Functional Walking Category:

2. 10MWT

Results: AFO traversed 4 m in 15 sec taking 13 steps

STRIDE CHARACTERISTICS: AFO AT SELF-SELECTED SPEED		
Gait speed		% N*
Cadence		% N*
Stride length (R)		% N*
*Waters; normal values for adult women		

Perry's Functional Walking Category:

ICF Domain: Body Function (Impairment Measures)

1. Muscle Strength (Manual Muscle Test [MMT]; 3/2/2016) Per Clinic Notes

MUSCLE GROUP	LEFT (REFERENCE LIMB)	RIGHT
Hip		
Hip flexors	2-/5	3+/5
Hip extensors	3-/5	4/5
Hip abductors	2-/5	4/5
Knee		
Knee extensors	3-/5	4-/5
Ankle		
Anterior tibialis	0/5	3/5
Extensor hallucis longus	0/5	2/5
Extensor digitorum longus	0/5	2/5
Plantar flexors	1/5	2/5
Ankle evertors	0/5	3/5
Ankle invertors	0/5	3/5

2. Spasticity: + Clonus in left Calf

3. Sensory Testing:

- Proprioception: Impaired at the knee and ankle
- Vibration, temperature, and sharp/dull sensation absent below T4 level

Precautions: Orthostatic Hypotension

ICF Domain: Activity (Per Clinic Evaluation 3/2/2016)

1. Timed Up and Go (TUG): 26 sec (fall risk)

2. 6-Minute Walk Test (6MWT; with SPC and AFO): 101 m (15% Normal)

3. Lower Extremity Functional Scale (LEFS): 52.5/80 = 65.6%

Examiner:

Print Name: Janet M. Adams, PT   Date: 4/23/2016   License: CA PT 11023

Signature: *Janet M. Adams, PT*

Examiner:

Print Name: Kay Cerny, PT   Date: 4/23/2016   License: CA PT 558

Signature: *Kay Cerny, PT*

Please see videos on the accompanying website at

www.healio.com/books/oga

Case Study 006

History and Evaluation

Patient/Client's Name: CS 006   **Gender:** Male   **DOB:** 07/23/1952   **Age:** 63

Gait Evaluation Date: 4/26/2016   **Ht:** 1.73 m   **Wt:** 218 lb

Medical Diagnosis: Inflammatory myopathy with vacuoles, aggregates, and mitochondrial pathology (IM-VAMP)

Onset Date: Spring 2015

Guide to PT Practice Pattern:

4C: Impaired muscle performance associated with acquired immune deficiency disorder

History:

Client 006 is a 63-year-old man with progressive weakness and atrophy of the upper extremity (UE) and lower extremity (LE), which began approximately 1 year ago. He has had several MD consults and biopsies with the most recent report (Keck Hospital of University of Southern California [Los Angeles, California] dated 1/25/16) indicating chronic denervation consistent with IM-VAMP. He walks independently with a tripod based cane for approximately 100 yards before fatiguing. He has significant UE and LE weakness and atrophy (left side more involved than right). He lives alone in a second floor apartment with 18 stairs that he reports he can ascend and descend independently by side-stepping using hand rails. He is employed full-time as an insurance agent and drives 50 to 100 miles a day to consult with clients. He states he is independent in all activities of daily living (ADL). He has difficulty manipulating objects with his left hand and lacks intrinsic strength with significant atrophy present. His goals include improving walking endurance, strength, and left UE function so that he can continue his employment and travel.

Past Medical History:

Hypertension and sleep apnea

Adams JM, Cerny K.
Observational Gait Analysis: A Visual Guide (pp 201-204).
© 2018 SLACK Incorporated.

SUMMARY OF GAIT DEVIATIONS

Reference Limb: Left LE

Condition: Barefoot with tripod based cane held in right hand

Essential Accomplishments

Weight Acceptance (Initial Contact and Loading Response):

Single Limb Support (Mid Stance and Terminal Stance):

Swing Limb Advancement (Pre-Swing, Initial Swing, Mid Swing, and Terminal Swing):

Upper Extremity (Reciprocal Arm Swing):

Foot/Floor Contact Pattern (Barefoot):

EVALUATION RESULTS

ICF Domain: Activity

1. 10-Meter Walk Test (10MWT)

Barefoot with cane held in right UE

Results: traversed 4 m in 7.5 sec taking 9 steps

STRIDE CHARACTERISTICS: BAREFOOT AT SELF-SELECTED SPEED		
Gait speed		% N*
Cadence		% N*
Stride length (R)		% N*
*Waters; normal values for senior men ages 60 to 80 years		

Perry's Functional Walking Category:

ICF Domain: Body Function (Impairment Measures)

1. Muscle Strength (Manual Muscle Test [MMT])

MUSCLE GROUP	LEFT (MORE INVOLVED)	RIGHT
Hip flexors	2+/5	3+/5
Hip extensors	2/5	2+/5
Hip abductors	2+/5	4-/5
Knee extensors	2+/5	3-/5
Anterior tibialis	1/5	2-/5
Extensor hallucis longus	1/5	3+/5
Extensor digitorum longus	2-/5	4/5
Soleus/gastrocnemius	1/5	2+/5
Fibularis longus and brevis	3/5	4/5
Posterior tibialis	4/5	4/5
Flexor hallucis longus	3+/5	4/5
Flexor digitorum longus	4/5	4/5

Significant atrophy in LE (left > right)

2. Passive Range of Motion (PROM)

JOINT/MOTION	LEFT	RIGHT
Hip flexion	25/125 degrees	30/125 degrees
Hip extension	-25 degrees	-30 degrees
Hip abduction	WNL	WNL
Knee extension	0/10 degrees	0/15 degrees
Knee flexion	10/0/140 degrees	15/0/140 degrees
Dorsiflexion	-10 degrees nonweightbearing (NWB) with knee extended	-10 degrees NWB with knee extended
Plantar flexion	WNL	WNL

3. Sensory Testing

- Light touch intact throughout peripheral and dermatomal distributions
- Proprioception is intact bilaterally

4. Girth and Skin Integrity

- Pitting edema in ankles (left > right)
- Marked bruising on anterior shins bilaterally

Additional Recommendations

ICF Domain: Activity

1. 6-Minute Walk Test (6MWT)
2. Functional Gait Assessment (FGA)
3. Lower Extremity Functional Scale (LEFS)

ICF Domain: Participation

1. 36-Item Short Form Survey (SF-36)

Examiner:

Print Name: Janet M. Adams, PT   Date: 4/23/2016   License: CA PT 11023

Signature: *Janet M. Adams, PT*

Examiner:

Print Name: Kay Cerny, PT   Date : 4/23/2016   License: CA PT 558

Signature: *Kay Cerny, PT*

Please see videos on the accompanying website at

www.healio.com/books/oga

Case Study 007

History and Evaluation

Patient/Client's Name: CS 007   **Gender:** Female   **DOB:** 02/27/1954   **Age:** 62

Gait Evaluation Date: 7/18/2016

Medical Diagnosis: Limb girdle muscular dystrophy (LGMD)

Onset Date: Inherited disorder with symptom onset at 6 years of age.

Guide to PT Practice Pattern:

4C: Impaired muscle performance associated muscular dystrophy (limb girdle)

History:

Client 007 is a 62-year-old woman diagnosed with LGMD at 6 years of age. She reports that both her mother and brother had the disease, as well as her grandmother, aunt, and uncle. She currently walks with contact guard assist, relying on a single-point cane held in the right hand for balance. She lives in a 1-story home with her partner who provides assistance with most activities of daily living (ADL). She relies on a power scooter (since 2008) for mobility in the home and community environment. She states she is able to walk approximately 100 feet before tiring, and is limited to the home environment or outside on level surfaces for exercise. She has both upper extremity (UE), spine, and lower extremity (LE) involvement with significant progressive weakness. She is able to achieve sit to stand with great difficulty pushing with her hands on her thighs, and then pushing on the scooter's chair arms to stand. She requires maximal assistance with dressing, bathing, and most ADL. She reports that the left side is weaker than the right and that she has significant anterior leg pain (right > left). (Right anterior leg pain VAS 9/10 and left VAS 2/10). She also described significant LE edema bilaterally when she is upright for more than 30 minutes. She does not use any LE orthoses.

Past Medical History:

Progressive weakness of all voluntary muscles for the past 50 years. She does not report any cardiac or respiratory problems.

Adams JM, Cerny K.
Observational Gait Analysis: A Visual Guide (pp 205-210).
© 2018 SLACK Incorporated.

SUMMARY OF GAIT DEVIATIONS

Reference Limb: Right LE

Condition: Barefoot with SPC held in right hand

Essential Accomplishments

Weight Acceptance (Initial Contact and Loading Response):

Single Limb Support (Mid Stance and Terminal Stance):

Swing Limb Advancement (Pre-Swing, Initial Swing, Mid Swing, and Terminal Swing):

Upper Extremity (Reciprocal Arm Swing):

Foot/Floor Contact Pattern (Barefoot):

EVALUATION RESULTS

ICF Domain: Activity

1. 10-Meter Walk Test (10MWT)

Results: traversed 6 m in 13 sec taking 18 steps

STRIDE CHARACTERISTICS: BAREFOOT AT SELF-SELECTED SPEED		
Gait speed		% N*
Cadence		% N*
Stride length (R)		% N*
*Waters; normal values for senior women ages 60 to 80 years		

Perry's Functional Walking Category:

ICF Domain: Body Function (Impairment Measures)

1. Lower Extremity Strength (Manual Muscle Test [MMT])

MUSCLE GROUP	RIGHT (REFERENCE LIMB)	LEFT
Hip		
Hip flexors	3-/5	3-/5
Hip extensors	2/5	2/5
Hip abductors	3/5	3-/5
Hip adductors	2/5	2/5
Hip medial rotators	3+/5	3/5
Hip lateral rotators	3/5	3/5
Knee		
Knee extensors	3-/5	3-/5
Knee flexors	3+/5	3/5
Ankle		
Anterior tibialis	3+/5	4+/5
Extensor hallucis longus	5/5	4/5
Extensor digitorum longus	4/5	4/5
Fibularis longus	3/5	4/5
Fibularis brevis	3/5	4/5
Posterior tibialis	4+/5	4+/5
FHL	5/5	4/5
FDL	5/5	4/5
Soleus and gastrocnemius (knee extended)	2+/5	2+/5

2. Passive Range of Motion (PROM)

JOINT/MOTION	RIGHT (REFERNCE LIMB)	LEFT
Hip flexion	25/125 degrees	25/125 degrees
Hip extension	-25 degrees	-25 degrees
Hip abduction	WNL	WNL
Knee extension	-15 degrees	-20 degrees
Knee flexion	15/140 degrees	20/140 degrees
Dorsiflexion	-10 degrees NWB	-5 degrees NWB
Plantar flexion	WNL	WNL

3. Trunk/Spine Strength

JOINT/MOTION	MMT GRADE
Cervical flexion	3-/5
Cervical extension	3+/5
Trunk flexion	1/5
Trunk extension	1/5

4. Upper Extremity Strength (MMT)

MUSCLE STRENGTH (MMT)	RIGHT (MORE INVOLVED)	LEFT
Significant scapular weakness	< 3/5	< 3/5
Shoulder		
Flexion/ext/abd/add/LR/MR	< 3/5	< 3/5
Elbow		
Elbow extension: triceps	3-/5	3-/5
Elbow flexion: biceps	4-/5	3/5
Wrist		
Wrist extension	4/5	3+/5
Wrist flexion	3+	4/5
Extensor digitorum	3+/5	3+/5
Flexor digitorum superficialis	3/5	3/5
Flexor digitorum profundus	4/5	4/5
Thumb		
Abductor pollicis longus	3/5	3/5
Extensor pollicis brevis	4/5	3/5
Extensor pollicis longus	4/5	3/5
Flexor pollicis longus	4+/5	4+/5
Intrinsics		
Abductor pollicis brevis	4/5	4/5
Adductor pollicis	4/5	4/5
Opponens pollicis	4/5	3+/5
Flexor pollicis brevis	4+/5	4+/5
First dorsal interossei	First 4/5, fourth 3/5	First 5/5, fourth 4/5
Fourth dorsal interossei	3/5	3/5
Palmar interossei	3/5	3/5

5. Sensory Testing

- No sensory impairments

6. Girth and Skin Integrity

- Significant edema in ankles after ~ ½ hour of weightbearing activity

ICF Domain: Activity

1. 6-Minute Walk Test (6MWT)

ICF Domain: Participation

1. 36-Item Short Form Survey (SF-36)

Examiner:

Print Name: Janet M. Adams, PT   Date: 4/12/2016   License: CA PT 11023

Signature: *Janet M. Adams, PT*

Examiner:

Print Name: Kay Cerny, PT   Date: 4/12/2016   License: CA PT 558

Signature: *Kay Cerny, PT*

Please see videos on the accompanying website at

www.healio.com/books/oga

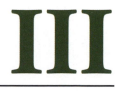

Appendices

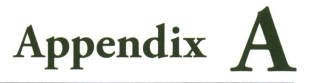

Appendix A

JAKC Observational Gait Analysis Form

Adams JM, Cerny K.
Observational Gait Analysis: A Visual Guide (pp 213-215).
© 2018 SLACK Incorporated.

JAKC's Observational Gait Analysis

Patient Name:		Gender: ☐ M ☐ F	DOB:		Date:
Medical Dx:		Onset:		Examiner:	
Orthotic/Prosthetic/AD:			Reference Limb: ☐ R ☐ L		

| | 0 | 12 | 31 | 50 | 62 | 75 | 87 | 100 |

		Stance				Swing		
Accomplish	**Weight Acceptance**		**Single Limb Support**		**Swing Limb Advancement**			
Phases	● **IC**	● **LR**	● **MSt**	● **TSt**	● **PSw** / ● **ISw**		● **MSw** / ● **TSw**	
Ankle	○ Fore Ft. ○ Flat Ft. ○ Abb HC ○ Inad. DF	○ Foot Slap ○ Inad. PF	○ Early Heel Off ○ Inadequate DF ○ Excess DF	○ No Heel Off	/ ○ Toe Drag ○ Inadequate DF ○ Contralateral Vault (PF)		○ Toe Drag /	
Calc	○ Excess Iv. ○ Excess Ev.	○ Excess Iv. ○ Excess Ev.	○ Excess Inversion ○ Excess Eversion		○ Excess Inversion			
Toes			○ Excess IP Flexion (Clawed)	○ Inadequate MTP X				
Knee	○ Inad. Ext.	○ Inad. Flexion ○ Varus	○ Inadequate Extension ○ Hyperextension ○ Extensor Thrust ○ Wobble ○ Thrust	○ Valgus	○ Inad. Flexion ○ Excess Flexion ○ Excess Contralateral Flexion		○ Inadequate Extension ○ Extensor Thrust	
Thigh	○ Inadequate Flexion ○ Excess Flexion		○ Inad. Extension ○ Medial Rotation ○ Lateral Rotation ○ Abduction ○ Adduction		○ Inad. Flexion ○ Excess Flexion ○ Medial Rotation ○ Lateral Rotation ○ Adduction ○ Circumduction			
Pelvis			○ Contralateral Drop >5° ○ Inad. Backward Rotation ○ Excess Backward Rotation ○ Excess Anterior Tilt		○ Ipsilateral Drop >5° ○ Inad. Forward Rotation ○ Excess Forward Rotation ○ Hike (>neutral) ○ Excess Posterior Tilt			
Trunk			○ Forward Lean ○ Backward Lean ○ Right Lean ○ Left Lean		○ Forward Lean ○ Backward Lean ○ Right Lean ○ Left Lean			

Developed by Jan Adams & Kay Cerny (JAKC) CSUN & CSULB
Illustrated by Daniel Sanchez PT

Summarize Deviations within Essential Accomplishments

Weight Acceptance:

Single Limb Support:

Swing Limb Advancement:

UE: Reciprocal Arm Swing   ☐ Yes   ☐ No

Calculate Stride Characteristics

Self-Selected Speed

Measure distance walked _____ (m),   Time to traverse distance_____(sec),   # of steps taken_____

Calculations:

- Velocity (m/min or m/sec) = Distance_____(m) / time (s) = _____ m/sec   _____ %N

    (x 60 sec/min) = _____ m/min

- Cadence (steps/minute) = #steps_____/ time(sec) x (60 sec/min) _____ steps/min   _____ %N

- Stride Length (meters) = Velocity_____(m/min) / ½ #steps/min_____= meters/stride   _____ %N

Note: 2 steps=1 stride   - therefore divide by ½ #steps per minute

---

Developed by Jan Adams & Kay Cerny (JAKC) CSUN & CSULB
Illustrated by Daniel Sanchez PT

Appendix B

Stride Characteristics for Adults Ages 20 to 59 Years

Adams JM, Cerny K.
Observational Gait Analysis: A Visual Guide (pp 217-218).
© 2018 SLACK Incorporated.

ADULTS (20 TO 59 YEARS)	VELOCITY (m/min) and (m/sec)			CADENCE (steps/min)			STRIDE LENGTH (m)		
	Normal (self-selected)	Slow	Fast	Normal (self-selected)	Slow	Fast	Normal (self-selected)	Slow	Fast
Female	77.67 m/min / 1.30 m/sec	37.01 m/min / 0.62 m/sec	99.36 m/min / 1.66 m/sec	117.59	67.61	137.03	1.319	0.891	1.237
Male	82 m/min / 1.37 m/sec	47.65 m/min / 0.79 m/sec	110.44 m/min / 1.84 m/sec	108.15	76.30	125.43	1.511	1.033	1.673
Total	80 m/min / 1.33 m/sec	42.76 m/min / 0.71 m/sec	105.57 m/min / 1.76 m/sec	112.55	72.31	130.53	1.422	0.967	1.470

Adapted from Waters RL, Lunsford BR, Perry J, Byrd R. Energy-speed relationship of walking: standard tables. *Journal of Orthopaedic Research.* 1988;6(2):215-222.

Stride Characteristics for Adults Ages 60 to 80 Years

Adams JM, Cerny K.
Observational Gait Analysis: A Visual Guide (pp 219-220).
© 2018 SLACK Incorporated.

ADULTS (60 TO 80 YEARS)	VELOCITY (m/min) and (m/sec)			CADENCE (steps/min)			STRIDE LENGTH (m)		
	Normal (self-selected)	Slow	Fast	Normal (self-selected)	Slow	Fast	Normal (self-selected)	Slow	Fast
Female	71.83 m/min / 1.20 m/sec	48.28 m/min / 0.80 m/sec	85.37 m/min / 1.42 m/sec	112.85	84.93	124.04	1.272	1.085	1.318
Male	76.64 m/min / 1.28 m/sec	49.64 m/min / 0.83 m/sec	96.71 m/min / 1.61 m/sec	105.85	78.92	118.69	1.450	1.159	1.630
Total	73.55 m/min / 1.23 m/sec	48.91 m/min / 0.82 m/sec	89.52 m/min / 1.49 m/sec	110.36	82.84	122.08	1.335	1.112	1.430

Adapted from Waters RL, Lunsford BR, Perry J, Byrd R. Energy-speed relationship of walking: standard tables. Journal of Orthopaedic Research. 1988;6(2):215-222.

Appendix D

Gait Analysis Report Rubric

Adams JM, Cerny K.
Observational Gait Analysis: A Visual Guide (pp 221-222).
© 2018 SLACK Incorporated.

NAMES: _____   Score_____/100

Gait Analysis Project Grading Rubric

Items with Points	Points Awarded				Comments
					Or (-) to subtract pts
A. Format, Completion, Organization, Signatures & grammar & language (8 points)	1	2	3	4	
A.1 Arial 12 Font, double spaced answers, organized clearly (according to template) with proper signatures (date & license) and any releases					
A.2 Uses grammatically correct, appropriate, culturally sensitive language throughout report					
B. Summary paragraph (4 points)	1	2	3	4	
B.1 Summary paragraph on current status (history with dates, dx, current & past level of function, etc) & gait deviation summary using appropriate, culturally sensitive language					
C. Discussion of Velocity, SL & Cadence in different Conditions Gait rite if available	2	4	6	8	
C.1 Table with Velocity, Cadence, Stride Length, SLS time (L/R), DLS time, FPA, Step/length ratio, with % normal for each, Compare different conditions (BF vs Shoe/brace) (8 pts)					
C.2 Discusses which determinants affect speed and compare conditions (brace vs barefoot) (Self-Selected Velocity, Cad, SL, SLS. DLS. FPA SL/LL ratios) (4 pts)	1	2	3	4	
D. Video Analysis (JAKC Form) Accuracy with Identified deviations checked or (lack of deviations-unchecked) (12 points total-2 pts each) For Barefoot/SS Condition	.5	1	1.5	2	
D.1 Trunk					
D.2 Pelvis					
D.3 Thigh					
D.4 Knee					
D.5 Ankle & STJ (Inv/Ev)					
D.7 Toes					
E. Gait Analysis with <u>probable cause</u> for each functional phase (36 points) (Include trunk, pelvis, thigh, knee, ankle, ST, toes as needed) For all conditions (BF/Brace/Shoe)	4	6	8	12	
E.1 Weight Acceptance (12 pts)					
E.2 Single Limb Support (Mid & Terminal Stance) (12 pts)					
E.3 Swing Limb Advancement (Pre Swing, Initial, Mid & Terminal Swing) (12 pts)					
F. Foot Floor Contact Pattern (4 pts)	1	2	3	4	
F.1 Accurately identifies foot floor contact pattern (& sequence) for each condition					
G. Tests to be performed (4 pts each) Using WHO language (Bullet List OK)	1	2	3	4	
G.1 Identifies tests to be performed to assess **"impairments"** in body function based on probable deviations & patient diagnosis					
G. 2 Identifies tests to be performed to assess **"activity limitations"** & **"participation restrictions"** based on psychometric properties (justify based on MDIC, reliability, validity etc) & patient diagnosis					
H. Goals & Treatments Ideas (4 goals with treatment ideas – 4 pts each) 16 pts total	1	2	3	4	
H.1 Goal 1: Identifies Impairment, quantifies goal, links goal to activity & participation measures, time frame.					
H.2 Goal 2: Identifies Impairment, quantifies goal, links goal to activity and participation measures, time frame.					
H.3 Goal 3: Identifies Impairment, quantifies goal, links goal to activity and participation measures, time frame.					
H.4 Goal 4: Identifies Impairment, quantifies goal, links goal to activity & participation measures, time frame.					

COMMENTS   **FINAL SCORE_____**

Financial Disclosures

Dr. Janet M. Adams has no financial or proprietary interest in the materials presented herein.

Dr. Kay Cerny has no financial or proprietary interest in the materials presented herein.

Dr. Olfat Mohamed has no financial or proprietary interest in the materials presented herein.

Index